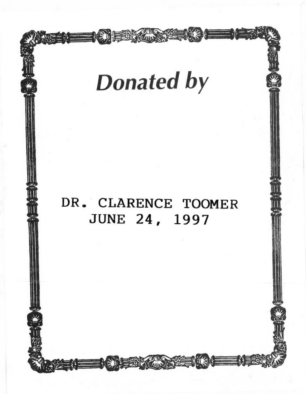

# The Private Lives
# and Professional Identity
# of Medical Students

# NEW OBSERVATIONS

*Howard S. Becker, series editor*

The close and detailed observation of social life provides a kind of knowledge that is indispensable to our understanding of society. In the spirit of Robert E. Park, the books in this series draw on an intimate acquaintance with their subjects to make important contributions to the development of sociological theory. They dig beneath the surface of conventional pieties to get at the real story, and thus produce ideas that take account of the realities of social life.

# The Private Lives
# and Professional Identity
# of Medical Students

### Robert S. Broadhead

Transaction Books
New Brunswick (U.S.A.) and London (U.K.)

**Library of Congress Cataloging in Publication Data**
Broadhead, Robert S., 1947-
   The private lives and professional identity of medical students
   Bibliography: p.
   Includes index.
   1. Medical students—Psychology. 2. Professional socialization. 3.
Medical education—Social aspects. 4. Medical students—United
States—Family relationships. 5. Medical students—United States—
Interviews. I. Title.
R737.B69 1983           305′.961           82-19502
ISBN: 0-87855-478-5 (cloth)

To Professor Leonard Schatzman,
*with gratitude for many things*

# Contents

Acknowledgments                                                    viii

Preface                                                              ix

1. Professional Socialization and Private Life                       1

2. Fashioning a Professional Identity                               15

3. The Impact of Professional Socialization on Students'
   Conception of Self                                               35

4. Private and Family Life in Professional Socialization            57

5. Private Lives and Professional Careers: Students'
   Management of the Future                                         75

6. The Impact of Private Life on Medical Training                   85

7. Conclusion                                                      101

Notes                                                             113

References                                                        115

Index                                                             125

# Acknowledgments

Since I began this research in 1974, I have become indebted to many individuals for their generous support and advice. I specifically wish to thank Mark Abrahamson, Patrick Biernacki, Odis E. Bigus, Kathleen Cahill, Fred Davis, Neil J. Facchinetti, Harvey A. Farberman, Barney G. Glaser, Oscar Grusky, Jerold Heiss, Marsha Rosenbaum, Leonard Schatzman, and Terri Wetle. I particularly want to thank Anselm L. Strauss, who chaired the committee which oversaw the research as a doctoral dissertation project; and Howard S. Becker, whose wise editorial counsel and strong encouragement guided the transformation of the dissertation into a book.

This study was partially supported by a University of California Regents Fellowship, a National Institutes of Health Research Award #HD00238 from the National Institute of Child Health and Human Development and #AG00022 from the National Institute on Aging, and a National Institute of Mental Health Postdoctoral Fellowship (USPHS-MH-14583). I also wish to thank the University of Connecticut Research Foundation for providing funds for having the manuscript typed and photocopied several times.

# Preface

This research was partly inspired by a contemporary physician who believed his thoughts about the medical profession were heretical. He therefore chose to disguise his identity by using a pseudonym, Dr. X, in a book-length confessional. The heresy Dr. X committed was revealing that he and his colleagues were human beings:

> Let me say that the cloistered existence of the doctor until well into his thirties makes him a late arrival in the Game of Life. . . . Inevitably, however, there comes a day when he understands, slowly at first, then more fully. But by then he has given too many hostages. He is no longer that pure entity, a doctor. He has become an impure mixture of husband, father, colleague and doctor whose responsibilities to others, whose commitments and promises have begun to outweigh the pure considerations of the healing science (Dr. X, 1965:19).

What attracted me to this passage was the image of a person as an "impure mixture," and the realization that what makes the mixture impure is the professional calling of medicine: *the* profession most dedicated to the normal growth and full development of persons. I found very quickly that the profession of medicine is not dedicated to the same principle for its practitioners and students, thus creating the conditions which lead to heresies and the need for pseudonyms. I also found that what makes medicine so zealously exclusionary of other priorities is not the practice of medicine but the profession. Becoming a professional can lead to major crises in becoming a person.

A review article on the collective well-being of physicians in the *New England Journal of Medicine* reported that:

> The suicide rate of physicians is two to three times that of the general population, equal in number to the loss of about two medical-school classes yearly. Alcoholism is at least as prevalent among physicians as in the general population, and under-reporting of physician-alcoholics is likely. Drug addiction may be 30 to 100 times more common among physicians than in the general population. . . . Retreat from family life is probably the most common adaptation to the demands of medical practice. A

progressive emotional separation from family life in the early years of practice becomes a *de facto* divorce (McCue, 1982:461).

These statistics lend strong support to my study—in a disappointing way. I found that medical training delivers a jarring blow to students' private lives and sensibilities: it inundates students for more than ten years, and in this time creates enormous socio-psychological and developmental deficits. As every action produces reaction, ten-plus years of slavish devotion to training (called "tyranny" by some) cultivate in students an adamancy to structure their professional practice so that they are eventually free of such problems. A determination grows, derived from the impact of training, to plan their professional future according to their private bidding. Such statistics are disappointing because they indicate that too many physicians ultimately fail in what they strive for as they leave medical school: a satisfying balance between professional and private life. The dilemmas students continue to face in becoming physicians is that the more professional they are, the more such a balance in behalf of private life smacks of relative failure and impure compromises in being a professional. As was emphasized in the *New England Journal of Medicine* review article: "Even physicians with reasonable working habits often praise colleagues who abandon their personal lives to their profession" (McCue, 1982:461).

# 1.
# Professional Socialization
# and Private Life

I began this study of the private lives of budding young professionals because the subject seemed so boring. From 1974 through 1978, I lived as a single parent and graduate student in a large married student community composed of medical, dental, pharmacy, and other allied health students. All of us were associated with a very expansive and prestigious medical university in California, though to my knowledge, I was the only budding young sociologist among them.

I became intrigued with the private lives in this community because from all outward appearances nothing much seemed to happen. In contrast to typical university communities, noted for their frivolity, wild functions, and robust social life, the action in this community was radically more subdued. During university sessions, which for most students included at least two summer quarters, weekends were conspicuously uneventful and offered little relief from the demands of training. Academic and clinical programs in medical centers are not effectively containable in weekdays only; they are notorious for consuming whole weeks. When there were breaks in training between quarters, students and their families left the community if they could. It was nice to get as far away as possible. In the meantime, the community itself struck one as a nonevent. Certainly the most active setting within the community was the children's playground. On the fringes of the playground one found spouses of medical and other health students, usually mothers but sometimes fathers, tending their children and biding time. For private life in medical school, biding time is the most characteristic feature. Private life takes the "back seat" to professional life in training. If one is a student's spouse, one's married and family life does too. Yes, a lot of speculation and planning for the future goes on, but in the meantime. . . .

The phrase captures it well: "in the meantime" refers to both that great *average* of time in private life left suspended in a virtual holding pattern, held in limbo until the envisioned payoff of graduation; and, for many students and their families, a time in private life experienced as *mean*, as in the notion among prison inmates of "doing your own time." Whether experienced as benign or malevolent, private and family life does "time" in professional training.

This is what captured my interest about the community: how do medical and other professionally aspiring students sustain a private and family life in the face of it being flooded by the voracious demands of training? Much like the children's playground, students' private and family lives were left to tend themselves beside the fringes of training. This is the most apparent impact of professional socialization on the private lives of students.

I also became interested in studying the private lives of budding young professionals because, due to the nature of my sociological training (acquired in a very small but vigorous graduate program situated in a niche of this sprawling medical center), I was trained to study everyday life as a phenomenon (see Douglas, 1970). Given the apparent orderliness, stability, and routine features of social reality—the unquestioned but questionable background of everyday life as Schutz (1967) said—I was trained to study fundamental sociological questions such as—how does everybody know what everybody knows? Or, how is the experience of social order achieved in conversation when people nod their heads in agreement to responses such as "you know," "et cetera," "blah, blah, blah," "dig," "and so on" (Garfinkel, 1967). In other words, I was trained to analyze the fundamental processes, procedures, and methods which lead individuals to experience everyday life as if it were mundane, routine, and ordinary. Given this perspective, in which the meaning of all objects and events in social life are seen as continuously achieved, they likewise become available for research. Even the most ordinary situations become problems in their own right, immensely fascinating and problematic.

I was intrigued with the private lives of professionally aspiring students precisely because of the ordinariness of private life. Here was a challenge to study everyday life as a phenomenon. Focusing on medical students and their families, I began to realize that the experience of "nothing much happening" in students' private and family lives *was* what was happening. Much of private and family life was "on ice," and people and whole families were forced into a holding pattern around the medical school, like airplanes in stormy weather, very much dependent on the decisions and scheduling of the control tower. Much of private life consisted of waiting, patiently coping, making do, and biding time. Except, as Barney Glaser observed in consultation, because students' private and family lives were seemingly so conscientious and quiet, so rationalized, scheduled, pragmatic, and sensible, "what we could be seeing here is a very slow burning fuse with a big bomb on the end of it. A bomb that can blow families apart because the wait turned out to be not worth it."

As it turned out, I did not witness many major blowups. Of the sixty medical students formally interviewed who were either married or single parents (out of a larger sample), two women students reported having been left by their husbands as soon as they had been accepted into medical school, and two other couples filed for divorce immediately following training during the students' internships. However, for medical students who get married while in training—approximately 65 percent by their senior year (U.S. Department of HEW, 1974)—what data are available indicate that physicians have very low divorce rates, even in comparison to other professional groups (Rosow and Rose, 1972). But in terms of the "slow fuse" hypothesis, the evidence also indicates that among physicians who divorce, the event usually occurs during middle age between thirty-five and forty-four. As Rosow and Rose (1972:592) concluded, rather than occurring immediately following graduation from medical school, "marriages break up considerably later than physicians suppose, when careers are already well-established and they are at the height of their professional powers."

While I did not witness many blowups, I did witness the fuse burning in various degrees of intensity, sometimes extremely. I studied the ways in which medical students and, if married, their spouses and families attempted to manage and control the *inundation* of their private lives with the largely nonnegotiable demands of professional training. I found that some students and their families were more ingenious and successful than others in managing the impact, as well as more conscious of what such management entailed.

In reviewing the literature on professional socialization I discovered that while existing theory is extensive and well developed, two important theoretical areas have been largely neglected. First, there is a conspicuous paucity of research and theory directly bearing on the impact of professional socialization on private and family life. Specifically, there is almost nothing on how the changes which the student undergoes in becoming a professional affect and relate to the multiple identities and relationships he shares with others. As Olesen and Whittaker (1968) observed, there have been a number of "thoughtful statements" by various educators and researchers on the relationship between the process of becoming a professional and fulfilling important "lateral roles," but no systematic or analytic study is yet available.

At most, there are a number of studies that correlate an assortment of variables (social class, religious affiliation, ethnicity, scholastic record) to predict student performance in medical school (see Fredricks and Mundy, 1976; Coombs and Vincent, 1971; U.S. Dept. of HEW, 1974). However, assuming that these variables represent multiple identities for any given person, there is no attempt in such analyses to specify the *meaning* of these other identities as they relate to the identity of being a medical student. This would provide some insight into the way individuals "symbolically" articulate one identity with another. Nor is there a discussion of how changes in one identity bring about changes in other primary identities. Finally, there are no analyses of the methods that individuals use to articulate these multiple identities with one another (see Feldman, 1979).[1] Existing studies tend to treat students as having a single identity, that of being *a* medical student. Their socialization experience is treated as leading to another specific identity, that of being *a* physician. A review of professional socialization research reveals a stark and fractured view of individuals. Previous analyses have ignored the manifold processes individuals use to organize their multiple identities into the coherence of a person.[2]

Second, in neglecting to examine the multiple identities which individuals embrace simultaneously, sociologists have focused on specific socialization processes and then analyzed them as if they prepared individuals for only one specific role and identity. As Davis and Olesen (1963:100) noted: "This has led to an unwitting depiction of career socialization as a uni-dimensional institutionally self-contained process in which the progress, travails and rewards of the aspirant are analyzed wholly within the context of the occupational role *per se*." On the other hand, the *meanings* and *purposes* of a given socialization process may vary immensely according to the meanings assigned by the individuals involved in it, as well as by the individuals officiating.[3] This would suggest that individuals are involved simultaneously in multiple socialization processes which prepare them for multiple roles and identities (Davis and Olesen, 1963). And, as was discovered in this study, that individuals interpret and use *specific* socialization processes as a means of preparing them for multiple identities and roles. A professional socialization process can be a means, at least in part, for individuals to fashion and express an assortment of multiple identities, and such a process can serve multiple ends. Existing research and theory on professional socialization have obscured the fact that, as individuals, students strive to become professionals as well as adults, men, women, spouses, parents, business people, and so on. In the case of medical students, their professional socialization was found to be an important means for them to realize and prepare for such multiple identities and pursuits.

In summary, the "finding" that students interpret and use their professional socialization to realize multiple identities and ends, calls into question the adequacy of past socialization research. It also calls into question the existing ideology of what "is" a professional. Namely, a central ideology of professionalism is that the practice of the profession is an end in itself. Professionals are described as a special breed of individuals, absorbed in the esoterica and specialization of their fields, intrinsically committed to fulfilling the larger mission of their professions. While this may be true, it is a half-truth. Professionals, and students studying to become professionals, see the practice of their profession as a means to a wide and rich assortment of other pursuits. Their extrinsic motives for practicing the profession are as compelling as any intrinsic motives. As Dr. X (1967:16) confessed: "Obviously, doctors are not boy scouts, nor are they deep-dyed dastardly villains. We are merely men living a system of man's creation that tends to give rather disastrously free license to each of us to fulfill our own needs—or greeds—regardless of the cost to others. In this the doctor is no less guilty than many of his patients."[4]

## Researching Private Life

The data upon which the following analysis is based were collected via conventional qualitative methodologies, primarily participant observation and formal interviewing.[5] As a resident of a university-housed community composed of medical and other health students, all of whom were either married or single parents, I was spared many of the problems which plague field researchers, particularly as participant observers. The problem posed by participant observation is negotiating a viable and legitimate social role for oneself within groups or organizations in which, as a social scientist, one is an outsider. What is required of the observer, as Olesen and Whittaker (1968) phrased it, is "making a livable world."

In formal organizations and institutions, creating a role for oneself is always tricky but can be negotiated in a straightforward manner. Given the public and/or formal character of organizations and institutions, a social scientist can always approach authorized officials and leaders, discuss his research interests and objectives, and attempt to formally negotiate a role which is unobtrusive and possibly even profitable to them (e.g., "free labor"). This is where it becomes critical: organizational "gatekeepers" are inevitably interested in something for nothing. The objective in openly negotiating is to ensure that the role one assumes is not so officially circumscribed that one's research autonomy is undermined. As Broadhead and Rist (1976:327) noted, "the pivotal concern for the gatekeeper is reciprocity, determined by what benefits the research can offer the agency as a whole, or the particular careers of the gatekeeper and other managers." To this end, in negotiating a role, participant observers must be intent on negotiating maximum access to informants, records, and observing areas, as well as freedom in data analysis and publication. While this may sound very complex—it is—much of it can be managed forthrightly in formal organizations and institutions because it is formally negotiable. What can be rationally struck between participant observers and gatekeepers is an equitable quid pro quo. The only danger, as Glazer (1972:11) noted, is that "the fieldworker will often promise things that he (or she) will come to regret."

In conducting participant observation research in individuals' private and family lives, the matter of negotiating a role for oneself cannot be resolved in such a straightforward manner. This is not to suggest that the matter of disclosing one's research interests is a problem; indeed, to conduct ethical research one must make full disclosures and secure respondents' informed consent (more will be said about this later). Making such disclosures need not be a major methodological obstacle (at least it was not found to be in this study). The much larger problem is first to conceive of a social role which one could "naturally" assume in persons' private and family lives, and then to negotiate it. Also, one cannot expect carte blanche access to "informants," records, observing areas, and so on. Married and family life—private life—has an exclusive quality about it in every personal situation. Even the prospects of a nonparticipant observer, silently positioned in persons' homes taking notes from morning until bedtime, presents a situation of extreme unreality and farce.

How, then, as a participant observer, does one "live" with others in researching private and family life, and yet not live with them? Certainly residing within a community is a first and possibly essential step, as Whyte (1943) and other field researchers have done. However, residency facilitates entrée into a community only to the extent that the community is geographically situated (given modern means of transportation and communication, many communities are not tied to geographical settings) and that community members "hang out" together, again, à la *Street Corner Society*. Few students and their spouses mill around apartment stoops and street corners in a medical university community. There are members who do hang out within such a community, although they happen to be between the ages of two and eight, and they hang out chronically. Since I was a single parent, it was by virtue of my daughter's relationship with these members that I came to "live" closely with at least twenty families of medical students over a period of four years.

Through these families I met scores of other families, many of which did not have children.

Due to necessity and convenience, parents quickly meet other parents through their children. And, because they share the responsibilities of tending children and keeping them busy, parents come to "live" together in many respects. This happens quite naturally, although it can be promoted if one cultivates the process, as I did. Such cultivation occurred in a number of ways, the most important being childcare. Being a single parent and a full-time graduate student, I relied on many parents in the community to have my daughter spend time with their children nearly every weekday. In return, on many evenings and weekends my apartment contained an extra child or two; such is quid pro quo for parents. Many parents, including myself, also belonged to a childcare co-op through which participants accumulated free time by tending one another's children. This amounted to an interparent support structure. Accompanying such an arrangement were innumerable favors and joint ventures: sharing cars, shuttling children to swimming and dance lessons, movies, excursions, birthday parties, covering for one another in times of emergency or hassle, lunches and dinners together, and so on. Because we came to rely on and help one another, we became friends. And friends share the mundane, day-to-day circumstances and problems of their lives. Such sharing happened most every day, in varying periods of time.

In the thick of this, my research interests began to gel. As I became more committed to the project, I began revealing to friends (as future respondents) the nature of the research and, much to my delight, they confirmed the importance of the research and expressed their willingness to participate in it. In an important sense, my reputation in the community became quite distinct because I was the only sociologist among these "medical marriages," and everyone who knew me knew that I was doing a study on the impact of professional socialization on private life. Thus, disclosing my research interests and securing informed consent was never a methodological problem; such disclosure validated my identity as well as opened doors and stimulated receptivity.

During the course of raising children, biding time, and "living" together, I talked with parents about family life in medical school. Most people naturally talk about private and family matters a great deal, and thus, such talk became an important source of data. Since I was also taking extensive field notes on what we talked about and analyzing those notes continuously (not during conversations, of course), my questions became more focused and organized. So too did my observations: of family timetables, divisions of labor and responsibility, routines, decision making, patterns of interaction, voiced concerns, problems and fears—all within the social context of medical training.

Eventually, in addition to the data being gathered through participant observation, it became imperative for more in-depth data to be collected through intensive interviews. For example, I was unable to explore some issues via participant observation simply because I could not gain entrée into particular settings. The data bearing on the process of facework in applying for medical school admissions, reported in chapter 2, were collected solely on the basis of formal and informal interviews. The data analyzed were of an ex post facto variety, consisting of reconstructions by medical students of the various stages and ways in which they attempted to organize an effective presentation of themselves. The interviews were focused on understanding how medical students conceptualized and interpreted the process of applying for admission to medical school, based on their own firsthand experience. The central problem in evaluating the adequacy of these data concerns the degree to which medical students' descriptions accurately portrayed the application process as they experienced it.

Since it was not possible to observe the admissions process directly, the accuracy of students' accounts was evaluated by the degree of similarity and overlap in the accounts of all students interviewed. Following the admonition to carry out a "constant comparison" in analyzing data, particularly by deliberately seeking out and investigating negative types of evidence (Glaser and Strauss, 1967), all accounts were first analyzed individually, seeking out and coding specific processes emphasized by each student. Some students were more articulate than others in recounting their experience. Each used slightly different words in describing various facets of what happened. However, in comparing students' accounts, while minor variations were noted, certain distinct stages and problems were commonly observed by all students interviewed. The accounts served to substantiate one another by isolating major stages and problems in the admission process. This led to the reasonable conclusion that the accounts taken collectively constituted an accurate qualitative description of the admission process itself.

In terms of interviewing students concerning the central focus of the research—the impact of professional socialization on private life—I began noting and comparing the great variety of private circumstances in which students found themselves: female versus male students, Chicano versus Black versus Chinese versus White Anglo students, single versus married students, single parents, female students who were pregnant while in training, older versus younger students, and all combinations thereof. Much of this initial substantive sampling was carried out on the basis of firsthand observations and informal interviews with scores of medical students and their spouses. I then began to assemble a comparative sample of medical students who were situated in, and represented, different types of personal circumstances. Formally, I interviewed forty married medical students and many of their spouses, each representing one or more of the different substantive categories listed above. I also formally interviewed twenty single students.

The interviews were usually an hour and a half long. Medical students are noted for their brightness. They found discussing their private lives rewarding, as most people probably would, simply because it is a topic seldom discussed in-depth with others, and yet is of maximum personal importance. Most medical students were candid in disclosing even the most private aspects of their lives and relationships with others—their worries, problems, frustrations, disappointments, hopes. In another sense, medical students responded as helpfully and eagerly as they did simply because, for many, sustaining a fulfilling private life while in training was a challenge, to say the least. To be interviewed in-depth concerning such very personal issues provided some students with an opportunity to reflect on their situation and understand it in greater detail.

The substance of both the formal and informal interviewing focused on two general problems. First, besides what data I was able to gather through published research on the nature of professional socialization, I also interviewed students concerning the nature of their involvement in medical school: what demands were placed on their lives, collectively, and what were their schedules, routines, and assorted problems in being medical students. Second, I interviewed students about the *meaning* of their professional socialization as it related to other aspects of their personal and private lives. For instance, I queried students on how becoming a professional relates to, as they saw it, being a woman, man, single parent, Chicano, adult, mother, father, and so on.

Simultaneously with the collection of interview data, I initiated the procedure of "open theoretical coding" (see Glaser, 1978). Such a procedure refers to the process of theoretically analyzing and notating the full range (but not amount) of events, problems, processes, characteristics, contexts, and subtleties of the substantive problems researched. Because the initial collection of data was not guided by predetermined theoretical codes and concepts, open coding involved applying, in a flexible way, numerous codes, vocabularies, and concepts found useful in theoretically rendering the data. With open coding, the language of existing theory became available as a potpourri of ideational counters, foils, and levers used to conceptually dissect the given problem. In the present study, open coding initially resulted in a hodgepodge of codes and concepts sitting curiously side by side. Eventually, open theoretical coding and comparison of codes resulted in the emergence of more central transcending codes and concepts.

For example, in coding the data on students' descriptions of the professional socialization process in medical school, there were a number of codes used to index the salient features of the process. Much of the data referred to the "nonnegotiable" aspects of the training, the "highly structured" and "unshareable" aspects of student involvement, the "high social value," the "uncertainty" and "risk," and the "unremitting workload." These codes and many others were frequently used in open coding, and they served to give dimension to the professional socialization process.

Ultimately, the code "inundation" was used to index data bearing on students' complaints that their private lives were being flooded and tyrannized by the training. (Barney Glaser first suggested the code in an analysis workshop.) Through comparison and reflection on the code inundation with all other codes dealing with professional socialization, I began to see two important connections. First, inundation was a collective problem of all students, as discussed in chapter 4. Second, inundation was a transcending concept because it subsumed all the other important codes—students' lives were inundated at times *because* of the "unremitting workload," the "inherent uncertainty," "risk," the "non-negotiable aspects of training," and so on.

Finally, two central codes emerged through open coding—inundation and articulation. The former code conceptually transcended the larger class of codes that provided a dimension to the features of the professional socialization process. The latter code conceptually transcended the class of codes that gave focus to how students saw their professional socialization as it related to their other primary identities, relationships with others, management of time and resources, and their adjustment to different situations.

At this stage of the research process, as the conceptual framework began to emerge, grounded in innumerable observations, descriptions, interview data, codes and notations from the field, and a survey of the relevant literature—the procedures of substantive sampling and open theoretical coding were displaced by the procedure of "theoretical sampling" (Glaser and Strauss, 1967). Future data were collected and analyzed with an eye toward further developing the properties, dimensions, and problems of the central concepts that emerged and "cored out" of extensive open coding and substantive sampling.

In returning to the field for the purpose of theoretical sampling, I attempted to gather more comparative data bearing on every concept and problem of the theoretical perspective which had emerged. In doing so, I revealed to the students interviewed the specific problems or issues under investigation. In this way, the validity of each particular theoretical point or assertion was directly put to the "test" in terms of its relevance, recognizability, and congruence with respect to students' own experience and reaction to the analysis. The research, therefore, by virtue of the procedure of theoretical sampling, became both progessively more developed and verified within the research process. By early 1978, I ceased theoretical sampling, sorted my field notes and memos into the framework of the perspective, and proceeded to write up the first draft.

## A Proposed Perspective

This is a study of the impact of professional socialization on the private and family lives of students. The impact itself is "brought home" to students by virtue of their involvement in training. Because the overwhelming institutional demands and imperatives of training are categorically applied to all students in any given cohort, students' orientation toward the training program tends to be collective (Becker et al., 1961; Shapiro, 1978). In facing such demands, students' potential latitude to organize all other identities, commitments, and relationships with others in private life is broad, negotiable, and individually variable. The ways in which students organize their private lives around their training and their emerging identities as professionals reveals both the impact of professional socialization and how it is managed. Such considerations constitute the major thrust of the analysis.

The first assumption of the perspective is that the impact of professional socialization on private life is *symbolically mediated*—it is a function of the interpretations and meanings held by students between their training and their private lives (Blumer, 1969). Much of what the impact consists of is negotiated among students themselves, both individually and collectively, and with important others (Strauss, 1978). The impact is analyzed as dependent on this array of meanings which students and others assign between involvement with training and outside relationships. For example, a married student's involvement in medical training could be perceived by his or her spouse as a simultaneous fulfillment of the student's identity and role as a spouse. At the other extreme, students or spouses could perceive such involvement as an obstruction or as unrelated to fulfilling a spouse's role. Assigned meanings of such a completely different nature would, in turn, be associated with differences in the impact of professional training on married life, producing different patterns of married life and activity, different types of identities as spouses, and different marital problems.

The second assumption is that the impact of professional socialization on private life is *reciprocal*—the training situation affects students' private and family lives, but students' private lives also affect and shape the training situation and students' involvement in it. Identities and relationships competing with the training situation can dialectically feed back into and redefine the situation itself. Adjustment to medical training is partially a process of students constructing the situation by introducing their own perspectives, both individually and collectively. Such perspectives are grounded in identities that derive from students' membership in groups and relationships outside of the training situation. They orient students to very different interests and issues in medicine, and result in varying types of group activities and priorities.

The final assumption of the perspective is that the impact of professional socialization on private life, and vice versa, is *dimensional*. Professional socialization affects students' conception of self and the multiple identities which, in phenomenological combination, they associate with themselves as unique persons. Professional socialization also affects students' relationships with others, particularly students' ability to fulfill the role obligations and commitments relationships require. The impact becomes particularly critical as it affects the personal resources, time, and energy students must divide between the voracious demands of training and the competing demands and responsibilities of private life. Finally, professional socialization affects students' personal visions of the future concerning themselves and their relationships with others. Medical careers have exceptionally long and distinct temporal trajectories (Glaser and Strauss, 1971) and students must continuously grapple with the problem of reconciling professional and private plans.

Reciprocally, students' private lives affect many different dimensions of professional training. Students draw upon private life as they shape their own commitments to training and their level of involvement in it. Students' private lives also shape interests in training, areas of specialization, and the geographic areas in which to pursue a residency and establish a professional practice. Lastly, students' private lives give rise to a variety of social scenes and associations within a medical training situation which may or may not have anything to do with the study of medicine. For example, besides a student culture, medical school settings also contain a number of alternative cultures, such as an athletic culture, an outdoor culture, and a free-form intellectual culture. Such cultures are derived from identities and interests students sustain in private life and socially cultivate with other members of a university community. In this sense, the competing identities individuals embrace in private life can redefine the nature of training and give rise to new situations within that setting.

In the following analysis, all the basic assumptions of the above perspective manifest themselves to varying degrees. This study represents the "flip side" of existing studies of professional socialization. The analytic focus is not concerned with exploring professional socialization per se or refining existing theory about socialization. Rather, it is concerned with analyzing the impact of professional socialization on private life, a largely unanalyzed problem to date. The study is concerned with revealing how students articulate their emerging identities as professionals with other primary identities such as those of "adult," "husband" or "wife," "mother" or "father," and so on which extend from relationships in private life.

The problem of articulating professional identity with private life begins with applying for admission to medical school. Chapter 2 explores the ways in which prospective students symbolically fashion a professional identity to gain admission. Through a strategic presentation of self, applicants make two essential claims to professionalism, which medical schools subsequently expect students to fulfill absolutely. First, in their demeanor, students make the claim that they already have a comfortable vision of themselves as professionals; and second, that there are no major obstacles in their private life to prevent their total immersion in training. The admission process thus foreshadows a number of enduring problems during training and beyond which students face in sustaining both claims. These involve major adjustments and sacrifices in students' private conceptions of themselves and in their commitments and relationships with others.

In chapter 3 the ways in which students symbolically articulate their identity as professionals with their more encompassing sense of personhood are analyzed. The reasons why such articulation is most problematic for students who are women, wives, and mothers are given, as well as for those students who view themselves as adults.

Chapter 4 studies the impact of professional socialization on family life, with specific attention to processes students and their families engage in to achieve a balanced family life. Attention is also given to the crises medical students face as spouses and parents in coping with the threat of family life being flooded by the overwhelming demands and priorities of training.

Chapter 5 focuses on the significance for private life which medical students hold toward the payoff of graduation, as well as how they manage the deflation they experience as that payoff becomes increasingly elusive. How students attempt to grapple with an uncertain future, and strike important compromises between their future professional careers and private lives, is then addressed. A growing determination emerges among students to structure important aspects of their professional careers according to their private bidding.

Chapter 6 analyzes the ways in which students' private lives shape the nature of their involvements and priorities in training. Given the multiple identities students embrace, an analysis is offered of the competing perspectives which accompany these identities, and how such perspectives serve, along with the "student perspective," to transform the training situation. The impact on medical training of "women's health perspective" is given special attention.

Chapter 7, the conclusion, provides a brief summary followed by an analysis of some unintended consequences of "punishment-centered" programs of socialization, as Moore (1970) calls them—medical training being one classic example. It also includes a discussion of the limitations of professionalism as that perspective governs the structure of medical training, and what steps may be taken in the future to bring about a socialization of the influence of professionalism on medicine.

# 2.
# Fashioning a Professional Identity

## Foreshadowing in the Admisisons Process

In applying for professional training, applicants are advised to appear to be already what they hope to become. For example, applicants to medical school, both in the written and interview stages of the admissions process, attempt to present themselves as budding young professionals, particularly in terms of personality, commitment, discipline, and sense of responsibility. At the very least, they attempt to present themselves as "high-grade ore," the stuff from which precious professional metals await merely to be extracted, refined, and polished.

Also, the objective of medical school applicants in the interview is to give the unequivocal impression that enduring the demands of training and becoming a professional pose no serious problems for them. Indeed, there is a certain genuineness in applicants' claim: while the practice of medicine is commonly portrayed as a "magnificent obsession," getting into medical school for most is simply an obsession, pure and simple. Once accepted, applicants assume that all subsequent problems of training will be manageable, if not matters of "small change."

Similarly, in the admissions interview, applicants do not see the matter of presenting themselves as professionals, eminently capable of fulfilling the expectations and demands of training, as a substantial problem. Such a presentation simply requires a bit of effective facework: applicants must dramatically convey through appearances, gestures, and uttered accounts an impression of themselves as ideal professional material (Goffman, 1959). For example, medical students retroactively speak of the "pitch" or "angle" they pursued in characterizing themselves a "professionals" before the admissions interview committee. Presenting oneself as a professional, within the brief admissions interview, certainly does not create an existential crisis about self; the presentational pitch is intended primarily for "openers," figuratively and literally speaking. As many students explained, getting into medical school is loaded with uncertainties. The objective is to hit the right combination in terms of one's presentation of self and the particular expectancies of the audience judging the performance.

15

Applicants consider the "pitch" and claims they make in the admissions process as preliminary to professional socialization. Once accepted, students view the real problems of medical training as directly related to learning the craft of medicine: absorbing mounds of facts and knowledge, passing formidable examinations, developing clinical skills, dealing with patients. Applicants see the problems they face in the admissions process as qualitatively different from, and largely secondary and tangential to, the central problems they will face in training. In terms of the orientation medical schools hold toward training, students are quite correct. As far as medical schools are concerned, such matters *are* secondary and tangential. Schools hold students' unequivocal assurances of their total availability for training as binding expectations to be taken for granted. The real problems of training are learning about medicine and developing clinical skills. In satisfying those demands, medical schools assume that students will act like young professionals and that no obstacles are in their way.

By its very design and structure, a medical school is oblivious to any competing priorities or needs other than its own. Concerning the training program, its contents, schedules, demands, and objectives, such matters are dealt with by the faculty and administration in a very protective manner for the exclusive good of medicine. Being charged as the keepers and executors of the "Holy Realm," those responsible are singularly committed to upholding and advancing the mission of medicine.

This exclusivity of focus and priority permeates the relationship of a medical school toward its students. Both morally and practically, the concern is to elicit 100 percent performance from each student. To this end, in screening and interviewing applicants, a medical school is intent on gaining the unequivocal assurance that students' private affairs will not be a hindrance to their total involvement and effort in training. *Pre-Med Journal* found, in a questionnaire administered to fifty-two American medical schools, that "at least one school interviews wives [and husbands?] of all accepted students in an effort to anticipate possible sources of future conflict and to obtain additional information regarding the personal characteristics of the husband students" (Ceithaml, 1968:53). Such intensive interviewing is conducted because, once the training begins, a school is not interested in dealing with excuses, exceptions, or problem situations deriving from students' private lives. A school is concerned that each student be in a position to assume total responsibility for his/her actions, and to perform in a way ideally commensurate with that of practicing physicians: in an independent, responsible, self-motivating capacity.

The essence and thrust of the socialization process in medical school is to yield the model professional who is idealized as a super individual in terms of autonomy, judgment, skills, commitment, and motivation. As such, the potential flexibility in working out special arrangements or individually tailored programs by students is extremely limited, particularly during the standard first two years of classroom training. Albeit, many medical students note that arranging special circumstances is more possible now than it was in the 1950s and 1960s (see Drake, 1978). Occasional course incompletes can be taken. Students can elect to graduate in five years instead of four. Student Affairs, Student Health, and various deans' offices are available for working out emergent difficulties such as illness, childcare or economic problems, schedule conflicts, and personal and family problems. Such difficulties are looked upon as extenuating circumstances. Special programs are not options afforded medical students as they characteristically are in graduate academic programs. Students are severely limited, particularly during the early years, to fashion their own programs, schedules, courses, and pace. Options for taking leaves of absence are only grudgingly granted.

Student orientation toward medical school does not naturally drift in the direction of flexibility and individual accommodation. Due to the high workload, the uncertainty of the pace and schedule (see Becker et al., 1961; Merton et al., 1957; Shapiro, 1978), and the moral, professional, and social attributes of the work, the student strains toward total involvement. When pressures and demands accumulate from either training or personal and family sources, students will invariably sacrifice or postpone nearly anything to stay in school and "on top of it." As one female student noted: "If there are conflicts that develop between my family and the medical school, inevitably the medical school wins. It depends on what the situation is, though. If I'm on call at the hospital, regardless of what happens at home, I'm going to be at the hospital. And that's just the way it is."

Students are very reluctant to approach the faculty requesting special considerations for fear of spoiling their hard-won success or casting themselves in a negative light. Arranging special considerations patently goes against the thrust of students' whole objective. The point is to appear "together" regardless of pressure or demands, to be in control at all times, and to invariably act "sharp" regardless of circumstances. Put simply, the standard against which all students are measured and toward which each one strives, is that of the ideal professional personified in every situation.

In the wake of the orientation sustained between students and medical school, what are regarded as secondary and tangential matters in the professional socialization process emerge as central and enduring problems in students' private lives and relationships. The professional facework students engaged in to gain medical school admission and their unequivocal preparedness to fulfill the demands of training, will have to be sustained throughout training and beyond. To do so, much more than simply facework as a remedy is required. Maintaining such claims about self and sustaining one's involvement in training, introduces a number of enduring problems whose resolution requires major adjustments, accommodations, and sacrifices in students' private conceptions of themselves and in their commitments and relationships with others.

The admissions process can be seen as encapsulating and thematically foreshadowing many of the enduring problems in private life which students must manage throughout professional socialization. Before examining in detail what these problems are and how students attempt to manage them, an analysis of the facework process in applying for admission to medical school will first be offered.

### Facework in Medical School Admissions

Individuals in everyday life are continuously in the process of embracing, presenting, and sustaining multiple identities (Feldman, 1979; Marks, 1977). Although they cannot "do" everything at once, phenomenologically and presentationally, they can "be" everything at once. Many identities are worn on people's "cuffs," as Goffman has said. One's age identity is relatively easy to assign within a general continuum ranging from childhood to old age. Ethnic and sexual identities are also visible. Speech accent frequently give away one's citizenship, geographic origin, and socioeconomic status. Individuals' names are revealing, as are clothing and general demeanor (Stone, 1962). As Goffman (1963) noted, individuals "give" and "give off" information, and the amount of information given off regarding one's identities is immense.

In primary relationships and among colleagues and friends, people generally like to be thought of in many different ways and are eager to drop cues to their identities, interests, biography, and opinions. It is in the revealing and sharing of such information about oneself that the deeper images of one's character, "essential" nature, and uniqueness are provided.

While individuals embrace many different identities simultaneously, the norms and expectations of different situations require them to presentationally emphasize some over others. Failure to articulate identities in ways appropriate to different situations can create many kinds of interaction problems. Many situations, particularly within formal organizations, call for only specific identities. Explicit presentation or expression of competing identities can result in either heightening the ambiguity of situations or disrupting interaction altogether. If presented inappropriately, different identities can introduce the suspicion of split loyalties and divided commitments, ulterior reasons, and signs of equivocation in one's perspective or position. "Surprises" as to who one is can be troublesome and threatening to others, causing confusion as well as possible embarrassment, discreditation, and shame (see Gross and Stone, 1964; Goffman, 1963, 1967).

For these reasons, one might expect to find individuals regularly hiding information as to who they are, yet the opposite is usually the case. Except for encounters between complete strangers or in dealings with con men, individuals tend to live out most of their lives, whether with friends, colleagues, or intimates, in what Glaser and Strauss (1964) would describe as "awareness contexts" that are relatively open or strive toward openness. This is because, as the testimonies of homosexuals have poignantly revealed, living a life of pretense and concealment is a trying and bitter business (see Cory and Leroy, 1963). The extent to which individuals live their lives as con men and "Machiavellians" has been overdrawn by some sociologists.[6] This is not to say that individuals never conceal portions of their lives, but that they prefer to live as openly as is comfortable for them, even frequently in the face of rejection. The problem individuals face is how to disclose information about themselves which may be secondary to a situation but primary to being deferentially treated like whole persons.

Similarly, medical students were found to be a very diverse lot, stereotypes notwithstanding. Any given student embraced many different identities simultaneously, none of which was necessarily more important than another. Many students noted that prior to applying to medical school they had led extremely varied lives. Attending college in the premed years provided opportunities for exploring and expressing many different identities and engaging in a wide variety of activities. Before they entered medical school, many students were employed in occupations unrelated to medicine. Also, many students were spouses and parents, and sometimes single parents. Finally, students expressed interests in a wide assortment of avocations, sports, and hobbies to which they were seriously committed (see Drake, 1978).

Students insisted that, due to the demands of medical school, applying for admission was one situation which required them to present themselves as if the sum total of their lives had led to and supported a single identity: medical student. As one student expressed: "In order to get in, you have to sell yourself that you will totally live medicine for the rest of your life, and that's all you want." To do so, students reported the necessity of presenting themselves as if everything in their prior and present lives had prepared them for the ultimate goal of becoming medical students. Applicants involved themselves in a complex facework process which evolved through four stages, each entailing a unique set of problems. These stages came to be designated as (1) anticipatory identification, (2) categorical identification, (3) individuation, and (4) normalization.

*Anticipatory Identification*

Medical students indicated that the first stage commenced years prior to their actual application, when they began to search out, on the basis of research, counseling, advice, and rumor, the criteria that medical schools use to identify promising candidates for medical training. As students learned the criteria over time, they began to invest themselves through formal training and study with the necessary prerequisite skills, experience, and credentials. As one student expressed:

> First you have to read everything that is available to you, and then you begin to see the kind of thing that they are looking for. You visualize it in terms of grade point averages, test scores, and letters of recommendation. You have to realize that in order to get into medical school, presenting yourself *as yourself* is the last step in the process. You must first think of yourself as a piece of paper that they're going to be looking at, and they can either throw it away or keep it.

Some students were more strategic in their efforts to gain admission than others, but all emphasized that the more deliberate and well organized an applicant, the greater the likelihood of success.

As students anticipated their application in terms of presenting themselves as an ideal medical student, they realized they had to make themselves identifiable in two different ways. First, on the basis of test scores, transcripts, GPAs, and the like, students were required to be identifiable on paper as a member of an aggregate. Later, in an admissions interview, each applicant was required to be identifiable both as a budding young professional and as a unique and substantial individual, two identities which should not be thought of as mutually exclusive.

*Categorical Identification*

The second stage involved students' presenting themselves on paper in such a way that they appeared as members of a categorical aggregate. Students emphasized that the objective at this stage was not to reveal one's uniquenesses or special attributes, but to display the attributes medical schools emphasize in determining the initial pool of serious candidates. Even in the "personal letter" that accompanies each application, students reported that there were several good reasons why, if they were to be strategic, they were reluctant to discuss any areas of their lives which did not directly contribute to the image of the aggregate.[7] For instance a third-year female student explained:

> I presented myself twice. The first time (in 1973) I had a Master's degree and my son was very young, and I was married. I presented myself as a woman who had always been interested in science, and who was going to be able to be a good mother, and do a good job in medicine. And I didn't get one interview, not even one! I presented myself really honestly: "I'm a woman who has worked hard, who has always been interested in science, and this is really important to me, and I'm going to show you how I can make medicine and my family fit together." My whole essay about myself talked about how I had worked out childcare so I could be a medical student, how I was going to be a good mother—and I didn't get one interview!
>
> So the next year, I became more serious and looked into how to play the game. I then didn't even include any mention of my son in the next essay, and I just presented myself as a scientist who had done research, but that I felt that clinical science was better for me. And I told them all this stuff about science, and more or less took the attitude that the only thing that they were concerned about was an image of the epitome of the perfect medical student and scientist. So I came on hard-core as a scientist, and more or less omitted any other aspect of my life.

A third-year male medical student was similarly strategic: "The one thing about the letter is that the theme was that I tried to integrate the technical and social aspects of my life. I said that I had all these technical skills and that I did well in science, but that I wanted some kind of social application. But I didn't discuss anything else, like my marriage or my private life."

Students reported that creating the identity of an aggregate member involved relating to all other potential applicants on the basis of attributes determined by the medical school admissions committee. However, just as survey researchers are hard pressed to locate their ideal American family, so too applicants can only approximate the ideal medical student, and even then in ways which may have little to do with their personal lives. Students reported that divulgence of the latter information, which still had to be selective and well articulated, had to wait until the third stage of the admissions process

*Individuation*

Articulation and selective revealment of students' personal identities and attributes occurred in an admissions interview. Now that one had been identified as falling within an initial admissions pool, students noted that the objective in this stage was to dissociate from the aggregate and emphasize one's individuality. It was time to take the offensive and make oneself look like a young professional, unique enough so that a lasting impression was preserved in the minds of committee members.

Analysis of students' accounts revealed that individuation was approached in two ways. First, students intentionally revealed a number of identities and attributes highlighting their uniqueness as a person, separate from the remaining aggregate of candidates. As one student explained:

> I knew when I went for my interview that I had to look unique. Many people would have excellent grades and test scores, and I knew I had to separate myself from that group. I needed to make myself look like I was something special. First you have to get yourself into the pool of serious considerations, and then attempt to separate yourself from them.

To this end, students reported that they revealed a number of identities, interests, and pursuits in addition to that of "medical student," such as being musicians, athletes, parents, members of various religious, political, and ethnic groups. For example, one student who had previously been a professional magician demonstrated his magic before interviewing committees:

> I pulled it out and said—"here it is." And I did that to make them aware that when I said I *was* a magician, that I really was. That I wasn't just a Mickey Mouse that had a few tricks, but that I really was what I said I was. And it made one realize that, for those people who interviewed me, I did something a little bit different, and they'll remember me by it.

Second, in order to individuate themselves, students reported that they revealed a number of identities and attributes which evidenced their deeper character and substance. As the latter student noted, medical school admissions committees are not interested in a "Mickey Mouse who has a few tricks." They are looking for persons who manifest an appreciable depth of experience and development, a demonstrated stability and productivity over a long period of time, and a realistic confidence in themselves. To emphasize character and substance, students attempted to express diversity in their biographies, past achievements, important responsibilities fulfilled, and present involvements and commitments. As one student explained: "It occurred to me that they would not be looking for someone that was absolutely centrally fixed on medicine. At the time I applied, I realized that the trend was heavily away from that.

The trend was more for people who were very well rounded and had a lot of interests outside of science." Another student said: "My pitch was that I was older, and that I had had a lot of experience—that I was an adult. That I've had a lot of experience in other areas than just going to school; I've been around just a little bit more. Plus, I have a family and I'm settled down in life. I'm steady, motivated, and for good reason!"

If individuation is to produce evidence of uniqueness, an in-depth and expansive presentation of self is required. This is not to suggest that students simply "let it all hang out," for successful individuation requires that information be shared, but in a controlled way (Goffman, 1963). However, the emphasis on individuation is definitely toward as much openness as is possible and effective. Given the orientation of admissions interviewers as gatekeepers into the profession of medicine, such presentation is expected to be in detail and "upon command," once the interview begins. Considering the importance of these meetings, applicants spoke of the anxiety which surfaced in having to face review committees composed of strangers and then, in a gush, divulging masses of information about their private and family lives. Each interview usually lasted less than an hour. Certainly with friends and associates, most applicants would have felt comfortable in sharing the same information, but over a longer period of time and on their own terms.

On the other hand, in the moment of an interview, a committee's task was to "get to know" each applicant as much as possible. For example, based on a questionnaire administered to fifty-two American medical schools, *Pre-Med Journal* advised applicants of the following:

> These medical schools added that they do not attempt to examine the entire character of the applicant during an interview, but instead they use interviews in conjunction with other information they receive about the applicant to determine character. In addition, individual schools mentioned that any gross deficiencies of the applicant's character will certainly be noted during a half-hour interview and that the success of an interview depends more upon the abilities of the interviewers than the amount of time spent during the interview (Ceithaml, 1968:55).

In addition, it was mentioned that, among other purposes (eight in all):

> The interview may also be used to detect gross deficiencies in personality and emotional stability, i.e., to assess superficially the mental health of the applicant. Where emotional problems were a consideration, the participants were in agreement that in such cases (and preferably only in such cases) the applicant should be referred to a psychiatrist for an extensive psychiatric interview (Ceithaml, 1968:53).

Students reported that committees frequently felt free to ask a series of penetrating questions quite unabashedly. For example, one medical student recalled: "I've even talked with women who were asked what mode of contraception they were planning on using in order to avoid motherhood while in training. And these kinds of issues seemed to be an area of fair game for women, but not for the men." As Lopate (1968:73) discovered in her research:

> The tradition of such questions has forewarned women applicants, and few are likely to be caught off-guard in their lack of "dedication." Some admissions officers have therefore come to design more tricky inquiries to elicit that elusive quality. "Where do you see yourself fifteen years from now?" the girl may suddenly be asked. On the other hand, the officer may inquire about her plans for babies, *not* wanting to hear that she sees her life as totally dedicated to medicine, but instead, testing whether she has a "normal" or "abnormal" set of needs and goals. A Dean admitted, "When a very feminine-looking gal comes in, I might wonder if she's fit for medicine." Thus, the girl applicant must play it both ways.

In the last fifteen years, because of the 1964 Civil Rights Act and other federal mandates prohibiting discrimination and infringement of persons' rights to privacy, stricter guidelines have been drafted by medical schools to limit review committees' lines of inquiry. Heretofore, committees had recognized no limits at all. Students expected to be asked just about anything. However, they emphasized that the objective of committees today is still the same: to gain as much insight about each applicant as possible. Several admissions counselors who were questioned explained that, although interviewers are issued guidelines, the large number of interviewers used each year by any given school makes compliance to guidelines difficult and problems occasionally arise.

Reciprocally, students emphasized that it was in their best interest to oblige an interview committee, to open up and respond briskly and enthusiastically. The objective was to appear trusting and trustworthy, confident and nondefensive—professional. Students noted that, after all, the objective was to give the impression that one had nothing to hide, and to make a lasting impression by emphasizing one's uniqueness and depth of character.

An applicant's uniqueness is presented through a disclosure of attributes and identities which go beyond the specific qualifications for medical training. In an admissions interview, this process of individuating oneself is accelerated and intensified. Some students reported that immediately following an interview they feared they had said too much; others that they had said too little. One student, who had been rejected one year following interviews at several schools, then gained admission the second year, recalled: "The problem that I had in the interview was not coming across forcefully, and that I really wanted to do this. And then I have a tendency when I meet people to be somewhat withdrawn, and wait and see where they're coming from before I open up. And the second year I applied it was the same thing—more rejections."

*Normalization*

In individuating oneself, each applicant faced one of two risks. The first was that, long after an interview, one's application was rejected for reasons that could not be determined. Following an interview, students explained they had no idea of how they had performed, or whether they could reasonably expect a letter of acceptance. A common expression from students was that interview committees held their "cards very close to their chests," so that applicants never knew the nature of the decisions made about them.

After receiving letters of rejection, students were left with the unavoidable impression that an interview committee had found something about them personally undesirable in relation to other applicants.[8] Knowing they had nominally shared equal status going into an interview, applicants who were then rejected found themselves searching for reasons why a committee saw them as less acceptable than other applicants— "Was it something I said?" "Did I reveal too much about myself, or too little?" "Was I too confident or passive, maybe?" and so on. All that students were left with was the knowledge that they had qualified for an interview on the basis of "objective" criteria. But, having presented themselves, a committee found something which made them appear less qualified than successful applicants. Thus the first risk in individuating oneself occurs after an interview. It involves being rejected because of some unknown factor about oneself in relation to other applicants, compounded by a lack of opportunity to mount a defense or make an appeal. One has no recourse and no firm knowledge of what has actually happened.

The second risk in individuating oneself involved being directly questioned or challenged about one's personhood. The risk was that committees saw certain identities or personal attributes as either questionable or incompatible with becoming a medical student. For example, some applicants identified themselves as "older students," others as "parents." Certainly both identities would seem to highlight one's uniqueness in relation to most other applicants, or to convey a certain substance and depth of character. Some students reported that admissions committees commonly focused on these two identities, as well as sexual and ethnic identities, with suspicion and doubt. Students would be challenged to explain whether they thought that, say, due to their older age and family responsibilities, becoming a medical student might not fit into their life in a workable way. Or in the case of single women, especially if they had expressed intentions to marry and have children, perhaps medical training was not a very logical or sensible endeavor, professionally speaking.

In individuating oneself, every personal identity or attribute revealed by an applicant could potentially be seen by an interview committee as questionable and problematic. This was the single most important reason why applicants were reluctant to divulge too much personal information in their application letter. Accordingly, in individuating oneself in an interview, the risk of being challenged over the "sensibility" or "feasibility" of what one professed to be and hoped to become forced each applicant to be prepared to *normalize* all possible "liabilities" into either irrelevancies, benign attributes, or positive assets. In normalizing, each student had to be prepared to explain how becoming a medical student was congruent with all other important identities and attributes he/she embraced. Normalization required applicants to reveal how becoming a medical student was symbolically and experientially congruent with the multiplicity of their respective lives.

For example, the professional magician was challenged in an interview to reveal how being a magician was relevant to becoming a physician. He explained that becoming proficient at any skilled endeavor revealed a lot about a person's motivation and creativity (i.e., character). He was no dilettante in magic, nor would he be in medicine. Second, in order to normalize his identity as a serious magician by revealing its symbolic connection with becoming a physician, the student told the interview committee: "There are certain fields in medicine where you can really break new ground, and this can be very enjoyable for you because you can really dream up the whole thing yourself, create the reality, which is a very satisfying thing. And the creation of new realities is the whole thing about magic, too."

In normalizing more mundane identities, many students noted that committees frequently regarded a student being female as a very questionable identity, particularly women who were also wives and mothers (see Lopate, 1968). For example, in a number of admissions interviews, one applicant attempted to establish the feasibility of being a woman, wife, mother, and medical student in the following way: "I tried to make the fact that I was a mother an advantage to me. That I had learned about caring for people. And that there was a certain amount of maturity that comes along with a marriage and a family. But generally, it was hard to use this as an advantage." Another woman revealed in greater detail why it was sometimes difficult to overcome the skepticism and doubts of some committees:

> I said, "I've had my children. I have proven my competence as a student while being a mother." And that I didn't see why having kids would get in the way. And basically, I implied that I was not going to be dropping out of school or out of medicine in order to have our children; that basically our family was complete. But listen, I was put on the defensive more than once by people saying, "You're going to drop out of school to have more kids," and I would say, "How can you say that! This is what I did *in* school while *having* my children." And they would point to other women who have dropped out of medicine to have children. And I said, "Well, I've already had my children."

The second risk students faced in individuating themselves was having the plausibility of their personhood thrown into question. Having advanced through the stages of anticipatory identification, categorical identification, and individuation, all potential students had to be prepared to normalize any identities and attributes unique to themselves. Successful normalization was achieved where students were able to convince an interview committee that they were unquestionably professional material, and that their endeavor to become a medical student was compatible with, and a developmental extension of, their private lives. To normalize skepticism, students were required to reveal how their interest in medicine fit into a much larger, cohesive web of other primary identities, commitments, and responsibilities, all of which were mutually supportive and integrated into the makings of a substantial person.

## Medical School Admissions and Private Life

Analysis of the facework process in medical school admissions foreshadows a number of central and enduring problems in private life that students find themselves having to manage continuously. Such problems derive largely from at least two major claims about self which students unequivocally assert in the admissions process—claims which medical schools hold students to with equal unequivocality.

First, students claim in the admissions process that they have a comfortable vision of themselves as aspiring young professionals and that they possess a genuine proclivity, personality, and temperament to naturally express themselves as such. Accompanying this claim is the corollary that their interest in medicine fits into a much larger, cohesive web of other primary identities, commitments, and responsibilities, all of which are mutually supportive.

The problems which emerge in attempting to sustain such a claim about self are extensive. Students confront them in the training situation and, even more profoundly, in their private lives. In the training situation the problems involved in sustaining one's claim to be a professional are managed by employing the same skills of facework and impression management which proved effective in the admissions process. In doing so, students experience a certain absurdity about themselves and other students in trying to sustain a convincing professional demeanor in the training situation.

For example, interviewing medical students about their sense of being professionals is always good for laughs—not at them, but with them. As Freidson and Lorber (1972) observed, everyone knows that physicians are supposed to be professionals, but what *is* a professional is a vaguely understood matter. Although they are aware of having to play constantly at being professionals while in training, medical students frequently sense a comic disparity between their private sense of self and feelings, and their propped-up professional demeanor. Certainly the disparity is not visible in observing student-physicians interacting with patients; nor is it visible when they are in the scrutinizing presence of medical faculty. During either moment, what an observer sees is professional facework in earnest. True, students' first dozen or so attempts at taking a medical history may take a couple of hours each; they may fasten the sphygmomanometer upside down occasionally, and take fifteen minutes to establish a reading; they may find themselves crumbling internally on every occasion in which they fumble around trying to get the right "feel" in a rectal examination; or they may feel more in need of tranquilizers for themselves than for the string of mothers they assist in delivery. But through it all, students sustain that look of cool competence, "affective neutrality," and objective poise. In such moments what one observes is the essence of budding professionalism.

In private moments with friends and family, the professional demeanor is abandoned with relief. Then one hears the stories: about being "pimped" by a resident following one's presentation of a case (being questioned unmercifully until one's knowledge is exhausted about a particular syndrome, thus forcing an "I don't know" response, followed by a "Well, why don't you know?") or being humiliated by a patient who wants to see the "real" doctor; being unable to skillfully curtail the irrelevant rambling of a patient about his private life and problems, never getting to the point of his medical complaint; a series of foul-ups and loss of confidence in performing any number of routine clinical procedures; or, the nearly sincere desire to strangle a screaming child who is definitely deserving of a prescribed shot in the ass, and so on. Objects of humor are frequently bizarre and sometimes appalling. Medical students find relief in deriding their own absurdity and pretension, as well as what they see in the behavior of patients, and other medical personnel.

In the training situation, the problems medical students experience in sustaining the claim of having a comfortable vision of themselves as professionals involve managing profound states of embarrassment and anxiety. Such problems emerge because medical students experience themselves as utterly incompetent, certainly throughout the bulk of four years of medical training and then some (see Light, 1980). Such feelings of embarrassment and anxiety are not unreasonable. In terms of the craft, medical students generally *are* incompetent. Accordingly, rather than having competence as young professionals, students must first fashion a "cloak of competence" that, they hope, will become less ephemeral in time. As Haas and Shaffir (1977:86) have aptly described:

> For those required to perform beyond their capacities, in order to be successful, there is the constant threat of breakdown or exposure. . . . Expectations of competence are dealt with by strategies of impression management, specifically, manipulation and concealment. Interactional competencies depend on convincing presentations and much of the professionalism requires the masking of insecurity and incompetence with the symbolic-interactional cloak of competence.

The observation that medical students' professionalism is a managed impression, a situated and provisional remedy for managing problems of embarrassment and high anxiety, also underscores that their "cloak of competence" is an essential means of defense. It is an important component of students' overall armamentarium for coping with the inevitable problems of uncertainty and risk associated with medical practice (Fox, 1957). It also helps reduce patients' reluctance and fear toward them as fledgling physicians for, indeed, students need patients in order to gain skill and confidence. As Shapiro (1978:62) observed:

> What is perhaps most frightening for students during this early exposure to clinical medicine is the possibility that they will not convey the impression of possessing at least some of the physician's competence. Were it not for their need to appear competent and professional to their patients, students would not be terrified about forgetting to review the musculoskeletal system when interviewing a patient, or about admitting that they cannot see the blood vessels when examining a patient's eye with an ophthalmoscope: a person has to learn some time.

Finally, sustaining a professional demeanor is essential to medical students and practicing physicians in order for them to enter private and sensitive areas with patients in a way that sustains a definition of public respectability and appropriateness. For example, in learning to perform a routine gynecological exam, such "behavior in private places," as Emerson (1970) described it, calls for a certain objective and detached poise to prevent a social breakdown on the part of everyone in the encounter. Any suggestion of inappropriateness in attitudes, gestures, or the setting itself can bring about cataclysmic reactions. The same need for professional demeanor is required in even less sensitive areas involving interaction with patients. Latent sexual overtones or suggestions must be controlled during routine medical histories or physical examinations.

Because of problems of embarrassment and anxiety, and as a means of defense, the claim of being a professional involves an identity with which medical students must seriously reckon. In the training situation, as in the admissions process, the central remedy used to manage the problems which derive from that claim are primarily techniques of facework and impression management. In private life, the problems which emerge in students' attempts to sustain the claim that they have a comfortable vision of themselves as aspiring young professionals run much deeper than managing problems of embarrassment and anxiety. Sustaining the claim requires effective facework and impression management while *in* the training situation, and the expenditure of enormous amounts of time, energy, and resources from private life to sustain each student's involvement in training. Given such expenditures, students' capacities to fulfill other primary identities and important relationships are severely limited or undermined. A variety of central and enduring problems thus emerge in private life which integrally derive from efforts to sustain claims of professionalism.

To begin with, sustaining such claims over many years, in the face of the overwhelming demands of medical school, involves expenditures from private life so consuming that students find themselves having to suspend or abandon many otherwise important identities, pursuits, and relationships indefinitely. For example, many students admire those among them who are single and without major responsibilities to others and thus in a position to collapse private life to a nub whenever necessary. Such sacrifices may be personally wretched, but much less vexing than those problems experienced by students who cannot afford to be so sacrificial. A considerable portion of students, those who are spouses, parents, single parents, and others in many varieties of personal circumstance, are simply unable to suspend certain important identities and relationships. As a result, in sustaining their professional involvement in medical school, many students find themselves in private life facing the problem of "hanging in there" as best they can, but chronically coming up short, severely compromised and compromising, guilt-ridden, and generally disappointed with themselves. These problems are exponentially compounded when students' feelings of inadequacy and disappointment about themselves are also felt about them by important others in private relationships. For example, it is one thing for a medical student who is also a father to feel guilty and inadequate about being unable to devote much time and energy to his wife and children. However, these problems compound if the student's wife and children feel just as strongly about his inadequacy and resent it openly. Important others can perceive the sacrifices students make in becoming a professional as made at their expense (see Marks, 1977).

Problems of inadequacy, lack of fulfillment, and compromised responsibilities can inflate in private relationships, leading to more intense problems for students, such as resentment and hostility from others, loss of moral and practical support, rejection, separation, and other calamities in interpersonal relations. The variety of problems which emerge in sustaining the claim that they have a comfortable vision of themselves as professionals reintroduces the same fundamental threat to personhood which students faced in the admissions process, but more profoundly. The criticism about their limited capacity or outright inability to fulfill other important relationships and primary identities forces students to again question the coherency of their personhood. Notwithstanding students' assurances in the admissions process, these problems pose the critical question of whether their involvement in professional training *does* fit into a much larger, cohesive web of other primary identities and relationships in private life.

Managing the impact of professional socialization requires students to *symbolically* resolve both for themselves and others how fashioning the identity of a professional—including all the required sacrifices—fits in with other important identities and relationships in private life. The question is, how do students come to *symbolically articulate* their emerging identity as professionals in relation to the multiple identities and relationships they share with others in important social contexts outside of medical training. These issues, as well as an analysis of articulation as a sociopsychological and interactional process, are examined in detail in chapter 3. The analysis leads to a reexamination of the internalization of professional identity and the "doctrinal conversion" medical students allegedly undergo in training.

The second claim students make in the admissions process that also foreshadows a number of problems in private life is that there are no major *practical* obstacles in private life preventing them from living up to the largely nonnegotiable demands of training. To sustain this claim, students have to resolve the many practical problems in private life that inevitably emerge once training commences. Such problems fall into three major categories. First, given the inundation with training, students must achieve a high level of *exemption* from private life. Just as persons must seek exemption from important responsibilities if they assume the "sick role" (Parsons, 1951), medical training requires students to seek exemption by appealing to the higher priorities associated with the profession of medicine.

Second, students' exemption from many relationships frequently requires some kind of *substitution* by others. As a practical problem, particularly in family life involving spouses and children, students' exemption from any number of activities and needs of the group requires others to take on these additional responsibilities. Inundation of the student's life leads to a highly focused kind of involvement toward medicine. Such specificity of involvement by the student necessitates a reciprocal diversification of involvement by remaining family members to meet those needs that would otherwise go wanting.

A final problem students must resolve to sustain the claim that there are no practical obstacles in private life obstructing their involvement in training concerns *scheduling* the plans and activities of private life around the highly demanding training schedule. Optimally, this scheduling calls for students to adjust their private plans and activities so they are inversely related to their training schedule. As with exemption and substitution, scheduling requires the approval and cooperation of important others in private life. Otherwise, private relationships become an immense countervailing obstacle to training.

*How* medical students routinely attempt to manage and resolve these three general categories of practical problems, foreshadowed in the admissions process, is examined in chapters 4 and 5. Students must continuously work on controlling and minimizing all competing demands, claims, and distractions in private life if there are to be no major obstacles in the way of training. As purely "management" problems, students must make adjustments in private life along the lines of minimizing, consolidating, and disattending. And they must do so in such a way that the adjustments themselves do not create additional problems and pressures in private life. For those students who must rely on the cooperation of others in private life, by exempting and substituting for them and scheduling their mutual lives at the convenience of training, successful adjustments are those involving a minimum of attention or effort. Optimal resolution of practical problems in private life means that students come to regard their relationships with others as "givens"— spontaneously and automatically adjusting to the overriding priorities and demands of medical training.

# 3.
# The Impact of Professional Socialization on Students' Conception of Self

## Symbolic Articulation of Professional Identity

Medical students must play at being a professional long before they become one and internalize a professional conception of themselves. The adolescent status implied in the title of Becker et al.'s (1961) classic, *Boys in White*, clearly conveys the developmental predicament of medical students. (As is discussed below, it is not uncommon for medical students to experience ambivalence in viewing themselves as adults.) Elsewhere, Becker (1964) offered a perspective on what is conventionally thought of as "adult development." He argued that development in adults consists not so much of "deep" personality and internal attribution changes, but "situated adjustments" by persons, frequently provisional and pragmatic, to the requirements of different situations in which they find themselves. As Becker (1964:41–44) explained:

> Many of the changes alleged to take place in adults do not take place at all. Or rather, a change occurs but an optical illusion causes the outside observer to see it as a change quite different in kind and magnitude from what it really is. . . . If we view situational adjustment as a major process of personal development, we must look to the character of the situation for the explanation of why people change as they do. We ask what there is in the situation that requires the person to act in a certain way or to hold certain beliefs. We do not ask what there is in him that requires the action or belief (see also Strauss, 1969; Becker and Strauss, 1956).

In analyzing the professional socialization of medical students, there is overwhelming evidence that the many transformations they exhibit during training are situated adjustments to the overwhelming demands and expectations of training. For example, as Becker et al. (1961:342) found:

> Students do not take on a professional role [and identity] while they are students, largely because the system they operate in does not allow them to do so. They are not doctors, and the recurring experiences of being

35

denied responsibility make it perfectly clear to them that they are not. Though they may occasionally, in fantasy, play at being doctors, they never mistake their fantasies for the fact.

For those students who internalize the conception of themselves as professionals or physicians, evidence indicates this happens late in the professional socialization process, and for many it happens only partially. For example in *The Student-Physician*, Huntington's (1957) research indicates that, throughout the first three years of medical school, over two-thirds of any given class of medical students do not think of themselves as professionals or doctors. Similarly, in Zabarenko and Zabarenko's (1978) study of "developmental stages in the growth of physicians," the growth of the physician identity was graphed as remaining both extremely low and constant until some period in the fourth year of training, followed by a sharp increase in self-identification (see also Fredricks and Mundy, 1976; Knight, 1973). However, both Huntington's (1957) and Zabarenko and Zabarenko's (1978) research clearly indicates that for a minority of medical students, even completion of the fourth year of training still does not lead to a strong sense of being a professional. Medical students "become" professionals throughout the bulk of training; but as a situated adjustment, the process consists more of facework and impression management than reorganization of self.

Eventually medical students do come to see themselves as professionals. While it may take some time to experience an internalization, students must manage their identity as professionals at the onset of training. They must act like professionals because of the expectations and responsibilities held toward them by others to do so. Becoming a professional physician involves acquiring certain clinical skills and mastering a body of accumulated knowledge concerning human physiology, biochemistry, and disease. It also involves a process of identity transformation which works itself out over a long period of time. Travisano (1970) provided a useful distinction between identity transformations that are either "alternations" or "conversions." Alternations involve an individual's appropriation of a new identity which is an addition or extension of prior identities: "These changes are logical; they are extensions or addenda to formerly established programs; they are cumulative identity sequences" (Travisano, 1970:603). As such, alternations "are relatively easily accomplished changes of life which do not involve a radical change in universe of discourse and informing aspect, but which are part of or grow out of existing programs of behaviors. . . . Little change is noticed by most of the person's others. There is no trauma" (Travisano, 1970:601).

Conversions, on the other hand, involve an individual's appropriation of an identity which necessitates or leads to a reformation and reorganization of prior identities: "Conversions are drastic changes in life. Such changes require a change in the 'informing aspect' of one's life and biography. Moreover, there must be a negation (often specifically forbidden) of some former identity. Conversion is signalled by a radical reorganization of identity, meaning and life" (Travisano, 1970:600).

Travisano's analysis emphasizes that the difference between a conversion and an alternation is determined by the extent to which a newly acquired identity is integrated and aligned with an individual's prior identities and biography. Alternation is a process of integration experienced as unproblematic, since it does not result in a qualitative reorganization of the relationships among already existing identities. Conversion involves the resolution of a major malintegration of a newly emerging identity with existing identities, requiring a qualitative reorganization of the relationships among them. The process may go so far as to require an entirely new constituency of identities. As Travisano (1970:602) explains: "The actor and all his others see his change as monumental and he is identified by himself and others as a new or different person. The actor has a new universe of discourse which negates the values and meanings of his old ones by exposing the 'fallacies' of their assumptions and reasoning."

In the case of medical students, Travisano's analysis underscores an interesting point. Regardless of whether the development of professional identity amounts to an alternation or conversion, either process requires students to relate, integrate, and align their emergent professional identity with all others. Whether doing so is difficult, traumatic, or totally reorganizing is an additional matter, although, as discussed below, the process varies greatly from one student to another. To achieve "symbolic articulation," as I will subsequently call it, the process may or may not involve a total reworking of the relationships among a person's existing identities. But the problem of articulation is fundamental to both processes.

In these respects, the term *internalization* refers to the process of medical students' coming to view themselves as professionals, and the world of medicine from the perspective of a professional, as in the notion of "doctrinal conversion" (see Hughes, 1958; Davis, 1968). Internalization also involves the equally profound experience of students' eventually striking a symbolic articulation of their emerging professional identity with their remaining multiple identities and relationships in private life. In addition, because such an identity transformation may be much more of a conversion than an alternation experience, involving considerable trauma, malintegration, and possible abandonment of other important identities and relationships, the difficulties involved in achieving a symbolic articulation of private and professional life may partially account for the length of the process.

To explore these issues fully, it is worthwhile to examine the nature of identity and symbolic articulation. The analysis can then move to an in-depth examination of the ways in which medical students were found to achieve a symbolic articulation of their emerging identity as professionals with the remainder of their multiple identities and relationships with others.

*Elements of Symbolic Articulation*

To have an identity is to be socially situated and assigned membership by self and others in a particular reference group, organization, social world, or "scene" (see Strauss, 1978a; Irwin, 1977). Identities are purely sociological phenomena, having no other derivation than the language uniquely created and used by humankind, which also gives rise to culture. An often quoted statement by Stone (1962:93) further elaborates what is meant by identity:

> Almost all writers using the term imply that identity establishes *what* and *where* the person is in social terms. It is not a substitute word for "self." Instead, when one has an identity, his is *situated*—that is, cast in the shape of a social object by the acknowledgment of his participation or membership in social relations. One's identity is established when others *place* him as a social object by assigning him the same words of identity that he appropriates for himself or *announces* (emphasis in original).

In addition to this conventional definition, to have an identity is also to have a perspective consisting of assumptions, definitions, attitudes, and values that individuals use as a frame of reference to organize and inform their thoughts and actions toward self and others (see Shibutani, 1955). As Foote (1951) emphasized some time ago, an identity provides an organizing and "motivating" frame of reference for oneself and others that partially establishes the initial definitions of a situation within which interaction occurs. Or as Stone (1962) also noted, in elaborating Foote's analysis, there must be an identification *of* one another's identity before an identification *with* one another can proceed. Frequently identification of one another is accomplished on the basis of nondiscursive symbols such as clothing, badges, location, and gestures—appearance. For instance, being a professional involves taking a particular perspective toward oneself in terms of how to act and carry oneself, how to appear in dress and demeanor, and a license to engage in special types of activities specific to one's occupation.

At most, the perspective which accompanies an identity provides only rough guidelines for how individuals should think, act, and appear toward self and others. Individuals can disagree over the particulars of a given identity, its perspective and prescriptions for conduct. Finally, many of the assumptions, definitions, attitudes, and values that make up the perspective of an identity can be called into question by individuals and deliberately changed.

For example, the identity of "woman" has been significantly called into question over the last decade by various women's groups. The result is that the perspective traditionally associated with the identity has become problematic, and guidelines on how a woman should "appear" and "act," in terms of vocation and emotional expression, are now much less definitive. As a third-year female student explained, the women's movement emphasizes that:

> Everyone should be the role that they feel comfortable in. Most women that I know feel like if a woman wants to be a housewife, and that's all they want, then that's great, just so it wasn't imposed on them. So I don't think there is a value judgment on them; you don't have to have a career to be a feminist if you are doing what you want to do. So now it's mostly fulfill your own potential rather than everyone has to have their own career.

For better or for worse—there is a range of opinion and controversy (see Lum, 1975; Andelin, 1963; Epstein, 1970)—what it means to be a woman in relation to the perspective traditionally associated with womanhood is now problematic *because* of the controversy itself. Women now have to carve out for themselves a female identity, and how they should relate to themselves and others emotionally, vocationally, and so on.

In addition to a perspective, an identity also carries social value— there is a hierarchy of prestige and importance among identities. For instance, newspapers frequently publish national surveys comparing the relative prestige accorded various occupational identities. Physicians, astronauts, and most professional groups rank very high, while politicians, government bureaucrats, and prostitutes rank much lower. Such a hierarchy of prestige also exists among devalued and low-status identities. For example, Tringo's (1970) research indicates that the identity of "old age" ranks below that of "blindman," "deaf mute," and "cancer victim," while it ranks above that of "epileptic" and "spastic." However, the social value of an identity can vary according to situations. For example, the identities of "medical student" and "physician" usually receive a higher social value than "homemaker" and "mother." Yet depending on the situation, the ranking can be reversed. As a fourth-year female student noted: "I don't get any 'goodies' at home for being a medical student. The kids could care less. All they know is that they need clean underpants."

Inasmuch as individuals simultaneously embrace multiple identities, they also embrace multiple perspectives on ways of relating to themselves and others, and each of these identities carries a different social value. Multiple identities symbolically articulate with one another in the way persons sort out the convergence and divergence of assumptions, definitions, attitudes, and values between the perspectives of different identities, as well as in the way they rank identities by assigning them different social values. Put analogously, individuals articulate multiple identities, symbolically, in the same way that social scientists and philosophers relate theoretical perspectives to one another, although not nearly as systematically. Individuals juxtapose, compare, and contrast the assumptions, definitions, attitudes, and values that make up the perspectives of various identities with one another. Individuals are capable of discussing the details of the symbolic relation of various identities, and they can specify problems that may obtain in the relationships among them. Because such problems emerge in attempting to articulate multiple identities, individuals become extremely conscious of the ways in which identities do or do not symbolically articulate with one another. In such instances, individuals face the problem of having to work out what could be called a "symbolic calculus" as to how problematic identities can be articulated with one another. Such a symbolic calculus eventually provides whatever degree of rhyme or reason that comes to exist, or needs to exist, between identities, and it provides the logic uniting an individual's multiple identities into the coherency of a person.

In these respects, individuals as persons are more phenomenologically "together" than social scientists have traditionally portrayed them. For instance, as Strauss (1969:152) noted: "Sociologists sometimes use the example of a man acting as a Christian on Sunday and a businessman on Monday, and they note that many men seem to be able to 'dissociate' or keep in watertight compartments the different role demands." In much the same way, Shibutani (1955:567) observed that individuals' lives are compartmentalized from one reference group to another, and that their many roles and identities are extremely different from one another: "Men have become so accustomed to this mode of life that they manage to conceive of themselves as reasonably consistent human beings in spite of this segmentalization and are generally not aware of the fact that their acts do not fit into a coherent pattern." Because individuals "conceive of themselves as reasonably consistent human beings," phenomenologically they *are*. The consistency and coherency of individuals in everyday life is not determined by the scientific rationality of an external observer, but by the interpretations of individuals themselves based on common-sense rationalities which govern everyday life "for all practical and reasonable purposes" (Garfinkel, 1960).

Except for people suffering from extreme types of mental illness or symbolic disembodiment (Laing, 1959), individuals do not view or experience themselves as dissociated, hypocritical, or schizophrenic. If they are asked—"How can you be both a Christian and a businessman?" they can reveal a symbolic *association* between the two identities. While individuals may belong to a multiplicity of groups, possibly partitioned from one another, the sum total of their lives is phenomenologically interrelated. The articulation of an individual's multiple identities is worked out in a symbolic calculus that determines, however problematically, the coherency and logic of the relationship between identities.

### Symbolic Calculi of Identity Articulation

Individuals embrace many different identities, and see and express themselves in many different ways. However, the specific meanings which interrelate their multiple identities are not objectively given. Nor are there any absolute rules for how certain identities must necessarily go together. In other words, why a woman also chooses to be a physician, Catholic, musician, spouse, or any other identity is not objectively apparent. The ways in which identities go together are problematic simply because the ways and reasons can vary immensely from one individual to another. To discover the nature of articulation, one has to discover how individuals symbolically relate one identity to another. The external observer must discover the meanings individuals assign in making up the symbolic calculus among identities, rather than imposing either their own reasons or even worse, asserting that, in "reality," individuals are phenomenologically dissociated beings.

Many students symbolically articulate their identities as women and medical students by integrating a number of themes which *they* see as shared between the two perspectives. Women who see themselves in feminist terms tend to view the themes of autonomy, competence, and individuality as integral to being both a professional and a woman. Women who see themselves in more traditional terms tend to view their involvement in a profession which is caring, nurturing, and directly involved in the reproduction of life as consonant with the traditional perspective of womanhood. As others have noted, the traditional relationship between being a woman and a healer has always overlapped considerably (see Ehrenreich, 1973). As one first-year female student noted:

> Women in medical school are able to express their femininity in terms of the way they are able to approach the patient, and their opportunity to care for people. I think women bring a tendency toward gentleness and tenderness, just in terms of physical things. Laying-on-of-hands kind of things that are needed, and that women seem to be able to do very easily.

Similarly, the medical student who was a professional magician had little difficulty explaining how the two identities related to one another. Indeed, many others have observed the parallels between the practice of magic in medicine and the practice of medicine in magic (see Kiev, 1964). The ways in which individuals articulate identities are not objectively given, but are problematic in the life of each individual. One must discover the meanings individuals themselves emphasize in bringing together multiple identities, and in articulating the perspectives and social values among them.

### Forms of Symbolic Calculi

While the specific meanings in the symbolic calculus between identities is problematic, there are a number of distinct forms that any given calculus takes. Identities are symbolically articulated in the form of a *blending calculus*, an *instrumental calculus*, a *diversionary calculus*, and a *problematic calculus*. A *blending calculus* involves symbolic articulation of two or more identities in such a way that they are seen as one and the same, or as evidence of one another. The quintessential example of a blended calculus occurs in the lives of many medical students who are also men, husbands, and fathers. Many married male students, and frequently their wives, see the student's involvement in medical school as a simultaneous fulfillment or expression of their identities and roles of being men, husbands, and fathers. The identity of being both a man and a medical student are commonly seen as blending easily. As a fourth-year female student noted: "I think that men are very sexy in their white coats and their ties, and that the doctor role is a very sexual, masculine role. And some men really turn on to that." Or as a male student expressed: "I feel sexier now than any time in my life. You know, you walk down the hall and women smile, sometimes rather seductively. I've never been treated that way before. I'm not even worried about going bald anymore, because you feel like you're a good catch anyway."

Similarly, many students who are husbands and fathers see their identity and involvement in medical school as *being* a husband and father. When queried about possible distinctions between one and the other, male students frequently found themselves somewhat dumbfounded at the question itself. As Epstein (1970:99) observed: "A man's duties and obligations *as a husband* fall primarily in the occupational sphere. If he earns an adequate living for his family, he has nearly fulfilled society's demands on him and, depending on his social rank, he has a wide range of acceptable behavior within which he may fulfill his other husband-father roles" (emphasis in original).

Being a medical student is frequently seen as a simultaneous expression of one's masculinity, and also as a husbandly thing to do. As to any conflicts, some students noted that the lack of time for being with one's wife and family is a real problem, but usually this does not call into question whether they are being good husbands or fathers. One student noted:

> My wife and her family are very supportive of my role as a medical student. In their value system, that is a good thing to be doing *as a husband*. As a husband, my wife obviously thinks that it's tough, but she doesn't think about the obligations that the school requires as divisive between us. There is no questioning my role as a husband. If it's absolutely necessary for me to be at the hospital for God knows how long, then it's absolutely necessary. I get absolutely no flack about my responsibilities in medicine, as long as there is a good reason for me to be doing it.

On the other hand, female students who are spouses and parents, inevitably find that their respective identities are not blended. As one fourth-year student noted: "A lot of the time when I am able to be home, I simply don't have the physical energy to respond to my husband and children in ways that I should. The thing is, men can be in this position, but they don't feel like they are not being good husbands. Men get the double 'goodies,' but women don't."

An *instrumental calculus* involves symbolic articulation of two or more identities in such a way that one identity is seen as a means of expressing other, relatively separate identities. For instance, many ethnic groups now see the opportunity for minority students to become professionals as a means of enhancing the social value of their culture and ethnicity. The appearance of increasing numbers of students who are Black or Chicano serves to dissolve the degrading stereotypes of various ethnic and racial groups, as well as providing the stimulus for increasing ethnic and racial pride and consciousness.

In addition, other social movements encourage their members to achieve professional status as a means of realizing the goals and philosophy of the movement itself. Most notably, the influx of women into professional education is a direct expression (along with other sentiments) of the women's liberation movement (see Epstein, 1970). Instrumentally, achieving the professional status of a doctor or lawyer is seen as a perfect "solution" for realizing the philosophy of feminism—that women are equal to men, that they should have the same opportunities and rights as men, that they deserve equal autonomy as individuals, and that they are as competent.

On a less grand scale, students see their identities as medical students, and eventually as physicians, as instrumental in supporting and expressing a number of other identities. For instance, many students see themselves as world travelers, and many who have a desire to live in other countries are attracted to the health professions because they are seen as offering geographically mobile careers. As one student expressed: "One good thing about being a physician is that if you go anywhere, there are reasons for you to do it, and if you ever want to practice, say, in Africa, then there's work there for you. In other words, you can visit a primitive society—I mean you can not only see it, but you can become a part of it." Or, as another student explained:

> I could well end up doing volunteer work in Mexico once a year, go down and spend a couple of weeks, or maybe a whole year. I mean, this isn't an escape thing with me. Last time I went down I had made plans to do a month's work of medicine, and then travel for two months. But I ended up doing medicine for practically the whole three months at this one clinic. So living in Mexico has gotten all wrapped up and really mixed in with what I want to do with medicine.

Finally, many students embrace a religious identity and are committed members of various religious faiths and organizations. Becoming a medical student, and eventually a physician, is seen as a religious calling. As Truman (1951:2) discussed:

> Religions contribute further, relating the powers and persons of the physician with the drive to do good; the high evaluation of the healing art is typified in Matthew 4:34: "And Jesus went about teaching, preaching the gospel, and healing all manner of disease and all manner of sickness among the people." We have here not only an identification of the act of healing with the conception of the ideal person, but an identification of the act of healing with the powers of the deity, both of which can be found in nearly all religions.

To gain admission to medical school, students articulate their multiple identities in such a way as to create the impression that being a medical student is the single most important identity to which they aspire. However, not only do students come to medical school with multiple identities, but inevitably they view professional socialization as supportive of fulfilling and expressing these other identities, particularly following training. Becker (1964) noted that the commitment of individuals to any endeavor is based on intrinsic and extrinsic reasons. Extrinsic reasons or "side bets" involve "linking of previously extraneous and irrelevant lines of action and sets of rewards to a particular line of action" (Becker, 1964:50).

In the case of medical students, undoubtedly the study of medicine is to some degree an absorbing and motivating experience in and of itself, as is earning the identity of physician. However, there are many reasons to become a physician (or a professional in any field) that are extrinsic to the practice of medicine.[9] For medical students, the professional socialization experience is seen in many ways as a springboard for the attainment of a number of widely varying rewards, pursuits, and identities. Due to the grueling experience of medical training, the "side bets" that students make as reasons to endure the process frequently become more compelling than the intrinsic reasons for doing so. As one third-year student noted in the "heat" of a particularly tyrannizing clerkship:

> I have a fantasy of traveling, and building a log cabin, and getting an old car and fixing it up, and getting a little ranch and some horses. And I think these fantasies are realistic. And I would say in fact that these things are *the* motivating factor right now in finishing school. They are going to carry me through the last stretch, and then when I get out, things are going to be good, and then I can relax.

Extrinsic reasons often supplant intrinsic ones because, in a way similar to the loss of idealism in medical school (see Eron, 1955; Christe and Merton, 1958; Becker and Greer, 1958), the study of medicine can be a disenchanting experience. As one anatomy Ph.D. student commented: "I always thought I wanted to be a doctor until I realized in graduate school how much I hate being around sick people." A third-year medical student expressed a similar feeling: "I originally expected to get more intrinsic rewards in dealing with patients. And now I find dealing with patients to be at times really frustrating, a lot more frustrating than I had imagined. A lot of problems you simply can't do anything about and yet the expectations are there for you to be able to solve them. It's pretty frustrating to admit that you can't help somebody, and to fail."

Thus, partially due to disenchantment, loss of idealism, and many other factors, students' investment in becoming a physician frequently becomes an investment to become something else, or to acquire something else. For instance, almost all students see medicine as a way to support the identity of themselves as adults, spouses, and parents. As one student expressed:

> Medicine is going to help because, when I'm through with training, I'm going to be able to have a resource that will allow me to do things that I'm interested in, particularly if I put my practice together in such a way. Thus, in ways, I can see medicine as a means to other ends, although not entirely. It's obviously important for me to develop a strong family, and I want to have a lot of time with them. I mean, medicine is supportive of this, although it depends on what specialty you choose. Some specialties are more amenable to having a family life.

Medical students see medicine as a means of achieving the *social* realization of identities as adults, an identity which they embrace sociopsychologically while in school, but which is socially undermined by their student status. (This issue is further analyzed below in this chapter.) Particularly for those individuals in medical school who have been students virtually all their lives, professional socialization is seen as a status passage to adulthood. They see medical training as a means to that stage in life where, socially, they finally achieve the status of adulthood with all the socioeconomic accompaniments and sense of independence that go with it.

A *diversionary calculus* involves the symbolic articulation of two or more identities in such a way that one identity provides an escape, or a respite, from other identities. As in avocations or hobbies, there may be no relationship between an individual's identity as a student and another identity, except that the latter provides the individual with a complete change in attitudes, emotions, and activities from those of being a student. For instance, when students were asked about the relationship between being medical students and skiers, golfers, tennis players, musicians, or a number of other identities, they typically answered that such identities represented opportunities to "get away." Of course, to "get away" or to "do something different" *is* a reason why individuals frequently assemble a number of competing identities. Individuals engage in different activities for the "hell of it" or "just for fun." If anything, such identities articulate with that of being a medical student by *not* relating to it.

Finally, although many identities articulate with one another in ways that are easily identifiable and problem-free, the symbolic articulation of other identities can remain continuously unresolved, perplexing, and incomplete. A *problematic calculus* involves the symbolic articulation of two or more identities in such a way that the relationship between them is, at best, partial and continuously shifting. In this sense, the perspectives among identities, or their social values, articulate in certain identifiable ways, yet there remain "issues" between them which conflict, contradict, or discredit one another. Their articulation amounts to a symbolic makeshift relationship of sorts, workable for the time being, or in specific situations, but fundamentally unsatisfactory and disturbing. For students in medical school, a problematic calculus frequently exists in articulating their identity of "student" with that of "adult." A problematic calculus frequently exists in articulating the identity of "woman" with that of "medical student" and eventually "physician." The problems and dilemmas of achieving a workable symbolic calculus among the identities of medical student, woman, and adult are examined in detail below.

## Medical Students as Women

Women have proven beyond a doubt that they can be competent medical students and physicians. As a consequence they are being admitted to most medical schools in increasing numbers. A nationwide study of health professionals revealed that "women studying for the M.D. degree have been increasing in both numbers and proportion admitted. In 1974–75, they comprised 22 percent of all admissions to medical schools, compared to 6 percent admitted in 1959–60" (Pennell and Slowell, 1975). This suggests that more and more women, particularly due to the women's liberation movement, have increasingly been able to symbolically articulate their identities as women with that of being medical students. The perspective that women have increasingly held toward themselves, of being equal to men in competence, competitiveness, and individuality, aligns easily with the perspective integral to being a medical student. Women have had increasing success in normalizing any lingering skepticism that has been held against them by virtue of their sex.

Having proved that they can be good medical students, they are having trouble proving to themselves and to others that medical students can be successful at being women, particularly in terms of fulfilling the expectations traditionally associated with that identity. This is due to a number of reasons. Many women find that being a medical student is a neutering experience. They discover that the expression of their femininity as medical students, in appearance and manner, is undermined by their medical student image. Glaser (in Lopate, 1968:73–74) reported that, from a survey of female medical students, there is "an ambivalence about being thought of as one of the boys . . . and then consequently, as a result of that identification, being thought of as less than a woman. They expressed vague anxiety about being a member of the third sex."

There are subtle kinds of institutional pressures in medical school that inhibit women from appearing to be anything other than "professionals." One student noted: "I have a new dress that I made, and I've been wanting to wear it for about two weeks, but I'm anxious about that because I am afraid that it's too feminine to wear on the ward. And I've put it on and taken it off. But it's real flowing and it's long, and it's dressy and new." This is not to suggest that some women do not dress femininely, but those who do sometimes experience a certain undercurrent of negative reactions toward them, even by other female students. One women commented: "There is one woman in our class who dresses very much like a fashion model. She will wear Chinese pajamas, and she's very attractive, and she dresses in a striking manner. And most of us think that she sticks out like a sore thumb. She just doesn't look serious. And she's a very flirtatious person, too. And thus she's talked about quite a bit by the women that I talk to."

Even more troubling is that many women see their medical socialization as turning them into men. As Campbell (1973:22) noted, "The 'culture' of the medical school apparently promotes the hypertrophy of certain (traditionally) 'male' attitudes and behaviors and often is supported by a men's club atmosphere." For instance, the demeanor of professionals as detached, emotionally unexpressive, and rational conforms more to a masculine image, and most physician roles are personified by men. A confirmation of this is illustrated in the experience described by a female student: "When I was younger, right when I was waiting to find out whether I had been accepted, I had a lot of dreams, and in all the dreams I was a man medical student! And I would wake up and I couldn't believe that I had had that dream, of being a man in a suit and a white coat. So I've definitely grown up in a culture where doctors are men." Another female medical student explained in more detail the "masculinizing" tendency in medical training:

Being a medical student definitely does not enhance one's femininity. I think there is a real threat of being turned into a man. And I don't know exactly what that means, except I'm turned into someone that is driven and compulsive as so many men are, and who doesn't have feelings or hasn't got sensitivity, and who just has no appreciation of beauty in the world. I feel really funny about whether I am dressing too femininely on the wards, and I try to be just as low-keyed as possible about what I am wearing.

In addition to the neutering if not masculinizing effect of professional socialization, many women have experienced their medical student identity as stigmatizing. This is particularly the case for female students who are single. First, being a medical student carries with it a very high social value or status. However, in comparison to the social status occupied by most men, such a high social status attached to a woman becomes a threat to men themselves. A woman whose occupational identity carries with it more social prestige and success than that of most men beats them at their own status game. And in the traditional battle between the sexes, men are notoriously poor losers. Many men feel so threatened by female medical students that they avoid getting involved in the first place. One student explained:

> The status difference between my being a medical student and most men really used to bother me. I would meet men that I was really interested in, and that were really neat, then the subject would come up, what did I do, what did they do, and as soon as it got established what my social status was, he would try to talk to me in a more intellectual kind of basis and try to impress me. And the whole relationship would just deteriorate because he wasn't being himself. And I'm speaking generally now—this has happened a number of times.

In reaction, many women try to hide their identity as medical students in private life. They pretend that they are "just students," nurses, or flight attendants, at least for the time being. This is because, on first acquaintances, if they reveal their true identity, many men then lie about theirs. As the student just quoted above continued to say: "You know, when they found out what I did, they'd say, 'Well, I'm a lawyer' or something, and it turned out later that they were salesmen or something, and they had never even been near a law school." As another student described: "I went through a period where I wouldn't tell people what I did. I told them that I was a secretary. And that worked fine, except I've been in situations where people would start making cracks about doctors and other professional people and I would start getting offended."

For most women, being stigmatized for being a medical student is a bewildering and disheartening experience. They note that male medical students are, as one student described, "in deee-mand! I mean, women get together and scheme on how to catch doctors." Yet women, particularly if they are single, almost always experience just the opposite. A third-year female student observed:

And I sit down and I watch, and I think, how come nobody is scheming on how to catch women doctors? I mean, everybody is avoiding us like the plague! And it's not just me. I've been in other hospitals and I've seen these interns and residents who are beautiful women, and it's the same story. I mean, we just get together in the cafeteria and we bemoan our fate. And *we* all agree that we've got good positive kinds of qualities, and that's what makes it all the harder because, what makes us proud of ourselves is what is hurting us. So whatever kind of social success there is is almost self-destructive.

Female medical students experience stigma because of the discrepancy between their occupational status and that of most men and, due to the demand structure of medical training, because they simply do not have the time to cultivate relationships with men. As one student described:

When I meet new friends, it's really hard to know what's going on. I don't have much time to really cultivate relationships, or to spend with people. I mean, medicine is a more demanding priority. And a lot of men say, "Look, men like a woman they can see during the week, and who is available to go away with him during the weekends, and can always do things with him and his friends. And when she says she's always busy, and when she's always saying that she has to study, when she's always on call, and she's never got time for you—who needs it!"

There are some very serious difficulties, therefore, which individuals experience in articulating their identities as medical students with being women. What articulation is achieved is continually problematic, and the symbolic calculus between the two identities remains at best partial, shifting, and provisional. Women have attempted to resolve the discrepant issues between the perspectives of the two identities in a number of ways.

First, although professional socialization in medical school strikes many women as a neutering experience, women have responded by reevaluating their identities as medical students, endeavoring to find ways in which their identities as women can be more effectively expressed. For instance, in discussing the neutering experience, one student commented: "I am finding that I am able to express my femininity in terms of the ways I am able to approach the patient, my ability to take care of people, and I think that means a lot. My ability to communicate with people. And I think that when you can come across with these added dimensions, you can really come across with an added rapport. And I know that this is an aspect of my femininity."

Some women refuse to alter their feminine appearance into the uniform, white jacket, and white shoes, even at the risk of being seen by others as unprofessional or out of place. As a female student described: "There are a number of women who come in and just look like dolls, and they always have, even when we were sitting in class. Obviously clothes and makeup and hair have always been very important to them. So although there is strong pressure there, I don't think being a medical student necessarily robs one of opportunities to express one's femininity."

Second, particularly single female students, attempt to avoid the experience of rejection by narrowing their list of acquaintances to only those who can appreciate and understand them. Such steps are frequently painful in that they involve the abandonment of former friendships and close acquaintances. Thus many women, particularly in their later years of training, associate almost entirely with other medical, dental, and graduate students whose occupational identities are of equal social value to their own and whose lives are equally constrained by demands on time and energy. However, as Lopate (1968:82) found, "for a minority of women who do not have outgoing personalities, the years of medical school can be extremely lonely, with few members of their sex as classmates and exclusion from total participation in the kinds of relaxation which unites male students. Even the most extroverted types will find themselves excluded at times."

Third, female medical students attempt to resolve the tensions between being medical students and women by rejecting the stereotype of what a woman "is," and thereby individuating their identities as women. As one female student put it: "There are all kinds of men, and there are all kinds of women, and people are just more or less sensitive to different things." By individuating their uniqueness, a number of the apparent conflicts and discrepancies between the identity of being a woman and a medical student apparently disappear. As Berger and Luckman (1967) emphasized, people are both products of social reality as it is given, and the architects of that reality. If problems arise in terms of symbolic conflicts within reality as given, one available solution is to transcend such problems by reexamining the assumptions of oneself and others at issue and recasting them. Women in medical school as well as women generally, have been seriously involved in the process of redefining the identity of "woman" for some considerable time now.

Fourth, most women attempt to resolve the dilemmas of being women and medical students by considering the possibility of choosing a career in medicine at the sacrifice of ever becoming a wife or mother (for those women who were previously so inclined). Some women apparently make the decision early on. For instance, one woman was interviewed for admission by a female surgeon who shared with the applicant what her experience had been: "The one woman who interviewed me was single and had been all of her life. We got to talking and she said that she never did have the time, and I believed her. She didn't feel that she could balance the demands of medicine and that of a husband and family, and she wanted eventually to be a top-notch surgeon." Or, as another woman explained:

> There are a lot of contradictions about being a medical student and a woman. Being a medical student means that I probably will never have a family. I'm 31 now, and I have three more years to finish getting my residency done, and then I'll be 35, and then, oh . . . I think it has a lot to do with socialization, too. Most of the women I've talked to in medical school have found it really difficult to establish relationships with men, especially for single women who are older. For another thing, once you're 30 and single, there aren't that many single men around. And then a lot of men don't like to go out with somebody in medicine because they don't want to put up with shitty schedules.

Most women probably postpone making such major decisions once and for all. However, they remain very much aware of the crosscurrents and dilemmas constituting their life and experience of self. Possibly such dilemmas cannot be solved while in training. Until later, then, women find themselves thinking of their recent past and imminent future with profound questions concerning the many different directions their lives may take. As one woman student explained: "I think back on it now, and if there were ever a choice, I would be a doctor before I would have a career as a mother or wife. It would be too bad never to have a family, but it would be even worse to have never had a career. At one time marriage and a family seemed so self-evident. Now I just don't know."

In articulating their identities as medical students and women, many deal with the problems of achieving a viable relationship between the two by simply living with the problems and ambiguities and looking forward to a change in the future. They become acutely aware of the issues attendant to being women and medical students and attempt to resolve them, but some problems are best managed by "putting on ice" and living with. Ambiguity is not the worst of all possible dilemmas for a person to face; boredom and the absence of ambiguity are probably worse (see Stone and Farberman, 1970). Thus a problematic calculus between one identity and another, while providing at least a workable, temporary articulation between the two, holds open the possibility of surprise and creativity in fashioning a more complete gestalt of one's life in the future.

## Medical Students as Adults

The years medical students spend in training constitute an ambiguous stage of life. Almost all students hold a perspective toward themselves as adults. However, being a student and economically dependent on a training institution or on parents (see U.S. Dept. of HEW, 1974), run contrary to adulthood. Chronologically and sociopsychologically, medical students have "arrived" as adults. They also evidence tremendous commitment to their work and conscientiousness toward themselves and others. They are responsible and capable of assuming heavy workloads and enduring considerable personal sacrifice. Many are spouses and parents, and some are single parents. In short, these are mature beings, perhaps inexperienced in worldly pursuits, but experienced educationally in science, medicine, and in other important matters such as hard work, responsibility, and commitment.

However, particularly in terms of their age, medical students, as Dr. X said, are "late arrivals in the Game of Life." Neugarten et al. (1965:711) noted: "Age norms and age expectations operate as prods or brakes upon behavior, in some instances hastening an event, in others, delaying it. Men and women are not only aware of the social clocks that operate in various areas of their lives, but they are aware also of their own timing and readily describe themselves as "early" or "late," or "on time" with regard to family and occupational events."

In terms of their age, medical students are both early and late in their arrival to the stage of adulthood. First, in terms of all the aforementioned characteristics (responsibility, commitment, etc.), medical students are early, particularly in view of their premed training. Moreover, the study of illness and disease, and the confrontation with serious illnesses, death, tragedy, and misfortune carry a considerable maturing effect. As one student noted:

> Your life becomes stricter because you have been given responsibilities that are far greater than most people's. Moreover, you have to adjust to seeing a very different side of people, mostly revolving around illness and death. What becomes commonplace to you, say, anal fissures, will gross the hell out of most people. That in itself requires a little more maturity than most people have. You have to learn to deal with it. And it matures you because it is a very sobering thing. And all the time you are going to medical school you are taking on more and more responsibility. So, in many ways, there's a kind of heightened sense of being an adult.

In other respects, medical students are late in their arrival to adulthood. Socially, medical students are denied the wherewithal while in school to live with the socioeconomic resources and sense of independence they associate with adulthood. For some, this impoverishment and dependency provokes tremendous feelings of frustration and powerlessness. In turn, such feelings become powerful motivating forces for students to finish school and get back into chronological step with their friends and peers in other occupations.

Even worse than the discrepancy between being an adult while lacking for many years the means to live as one, is the experience in medical school of being treated as if one were an adolescent—some say, like a child. Students feel that much of the training in medical school is based on a kind of insidious humiliation and intimidation. One student noted: "In the first two years of medical school, we were treated like third graders, and the information was just sort of poured on us, and we were supposed to memorize it and spit it back on the tests. And seldom were we even encouraged to think, or given any praise for thinking, and we definitely were not encouraged to think conceptually or independently." Similarly, a fourth-year student noted that being treated like a "third grader" applies to the clerkship years too:

> In this same rotation, where they are telling us that we should have the same responsibility as doctors, they then take roll at lectures! *They're taking roll!* And it's so degrading, you know. And they are filling up our time, as if we couldn't keep ourselves busy. For instance, today I had a patient that cancelled and they came in and wanted to know what I was doing with my time, like a kindergartener, so I wouldn't waste it. They take roll at lectures, as though we didn't care about learning medicine and had to have guilt induced into us; it's really disgusting.

Feelings of humiliation conveyed to students by medical school faculty and physicians are indirectly compounded by the inherent process of clerkship training. The effect of being moved to a new clerkship situation every four to six weeks can be disorienting and confusing, wherein students never feel secure in who they are, what they can or cannot do, or exactly how to do something, even if they know what is expected of them. As expressed by a fourth-year student: "I feel incompetent, confused, and dependent—that most people around me know more than I do, know the system better than I do. And especially with this clerkship business, whenever I get moved to a new scene, I feel totally lost again."

Professional socialization in medical school partially accelerates students' sense of being adults, yet in many ways prevents them from feeling or perceiving themselves as such. Accordingly, the ways in which students articulate their identity of medical student with that of adult is inevitably achieved on the basis of a problematic calculus. Such a calculus involves, first, an acceptance of the ambiguity between the two identities. Students are thereby able to symbolically acknowledge those aspects of being a medical student that tend to emphasize their sense of adulthood, e.g., the themes of responsibility, maturity in dealing with life and death issues, commitment, and competence.

Those aspects of being a medical student that tend to contradict their sense of adulthood must simply be tolerated. However, as discussed in chapter 5, such toleration is articulated in time. Professional socialization postpones students' sense of being adults, but it also becomes a solution to the problem. As a highly scheduled and regularized career trajectory (Glaser and Strauss, 1971), professional socialization becomes a status passage to achieving full adulthood. Until the completion of that passage, professional socialization serves as a socially validated alibi students use to neutralize the discrepancies of their being adults, yet "still just students" in mid-life.

# 4.
# Private and Family Life in Professional Socialization

Although individuals symbolically embrace multiple identities, many of those identities call for the enactment of roles and carrying out of responsibilities in order for them to be socially validated and sustained. For example, while bearing a child makes one a parent, neglect in carrying out the roles and responsibilities of that identity can call it into question. Due to lack of time, energy, emotions, and resources, the behavioral expression of some identities can become problematic or untenable (see Moore, 1963; French and Caplan, 1972). Thus, multiple identities must be *behaviorally articulated* with one another such that the wherewithal is managed sufficiently to permit the expression of competing identities, particularly those which are not simply worn on one's "cuff."

For medical students, notwithstanding their claim in the admissions process that there are no practical obstacles to their total involvement in training, the behavioral management of their lives is an immense problem. This is because students' involvement in medical school, given their high level of commitment (Marks, 1977), tends to inundate their lives and undermine the possibility of expressing competing identities and fulfilling relationships. For students who also happen to be spouses and parents, the inundation of their lives and relationships has an even greater impact.[10] Students, along with their significant others, must of necessity attempt to salvage whatever time, energy, emotions, and resources they can to fulfill their identities as individuals, spouses, and parents.

Below is presented an analysis of the structural conditions, such as workload, schedules, and priorities, which create and sustain the inundation of students' lives with medical training. An analysis of the impact of professional socialization on the family life of students who are spouses and parents then follows, with specific focus on the processes that students and their families engage in to achieve a balanced family life. The analysis concludes with an examination of medical students as spouses and parents, and the crises they commonly face in behaviorally articulating these identities with one another.

## Inundation of the Medical Student's Life

As a process, inundation refers to an individual's life being flooded and dominated by a substantively narrow set of concerns and rounds of activities. It involves the absorption and encapsulation of an individual's general range of identities, interests, and activities into a far more substantively focused order of events and concerns usually pivoting around a single, all-informing identity. As Coser (1974) described it, medical training is a type of "greedy institution," lacking any reluctance to tax all one's time, energy, emotions, and commitments. Lemert's (1951) analysis of societal reaction to deviant behavior examined how an individual's life prior to arrest becomes inundated with the overwhelming forces of criminal adjudication, incarceration, and stigmatization, resulting in a life and identity centrally organized around a life of crime.

Professional socialization can be conceived of as an equally profound societal reaction. Although embossed with a very esteemed ideology and purpose, commencement of medical training delivers a jarring blow to private life and subjective sensibilities. As Shapiro (1978:30) observed about himself and other medical students: "If students have been involved in extra-curricular activities as undergraduates, they rapidly dissociate themselves from the friendships and activities of premedical days; no more debating, no more work on the student newspaper, no more work on the film society, no more political activism." As an inundating experience, involvement in medical training is one of many substantive events which could be socially analyzed from a "societal reaction" perspective. As Lemert (1951:24) noted, "the behavior of the genius, the motion-picture star, the exceptionally beautiful woman, and the renowned athlete should lend itself to the same systematic analysis as that which is applied to the criminal, the pauper, or the sex delinquent."

For most medical students, becoming a doctor has been a "do or die" compulsion slowly kindling since early adolescence, further nurtured through years of grinding competitiveness, immersion in study, and immeasurable sacrifice. The obsession of some students to become doctors may be simply a conditioned "premed" attitude rooted extensively in personal identity and biography (see Levitt, 1966; Leif, 1971). Important criteria used by medical review committees in screening applicants are indices which reveal students' prior dedication, studiousness, and motivation over many years (see Best et al., 1974; Rosenberg, 1973).

Regardless of any predisposing tendencies that may underlie each applicant's absorption in becoming a medical student, whatever unremitting drive or ambition each student may bring to medical school is easily surpassed by the demands of medical training. The forces which promote the inundation of students' lives with medical training are not rooted so much in their personal psychology or in their early socialization—medical students are not as "inherently" obsessive-compulsive as some assert. As a "situated adjustment," much of their motivation is a response to the training situation in which they collectively find themselves. "Obsessive-compulsive" may more aptly describe the nature of the training situation than the students (see Becker, 1968). Similarly, the alleged characteristic cynicism of medical students while in training (Eron, 1955) has not been shown to be an inevitable personality attribute, but a provisional attitude situationally assumed largely in response to the clinical impotency and lack of responsibility allowed them in medical training (Becker and Geer, 1958). The forces promoting the inundation of students' lives with medical training are rooted in the professional socialization process itself.

The most apparent and immediate inundating condition faced by each medical student is a high-demand workload. The objective of medical training is to elicit maximum performance from each student, and the continual assignment of an immense workload both initiates and sustains the process. Medical students quickly discover that "you can never do all the work," and indeed the faculty typically forewarns each incoming cohort that "you'll never learn all that you need to know, and just get used to it." Regardless of the volume of work or energy expended in any given day, there is always more. As one student expressed: "If I was to do all of the work, and read all that was assigned, I would be at it twenty-four hours a day."

When it comes to the technique of studying, medical students are seasoned "pros." Regardless of the volume of work during midterms or finals, seldom do most medical students find themselves technically overloaded. Managing a workload is affected by a number of properties such as the skills, psychology, and previous educational experience of the student, as well as the number of competing problems to be managed outside of medical training. But it is not uncommon to discover students who claim that the workload in medical school is neither intellectually nor physically formidable. These students "pooh pooh" what they see as the lingering, high-anxiety "premed attitude" that many medical students continue to exhibit.

Irrespective of whether most students may find themselves pressed or overloaded, the sheer volume of work that must be faced each day requires continuous attention and of considerable quality. Some students find the workload exhilarating and a "snap," while others find it grueling and painstaking—it is a condition all students must continuously manage as best they can. It is an endlessly absorbing task (see Becker et al., 1961).

A second condition promoting the total immersion of students in medical training is its uncertain and risk-laden nature (Fox, 1957; Coser, 1979). Medical students complain of constantly "being on the spot," being caught off guard, having to face an endless number of exams and a myriad changing problems, situations, and expectations, as well as constant faculty criticism. Regarding the latter, students describe what they call "pimping" by faculty members:

> It's really incredible, because on rounds the staff will ask you questions that the students call "pimping." They will ask you questions, and they keep asking you questions until they make you feel about *this* high. They'll keep pushing you farther and farther until they've revealed the depth of your knowledge or the strength of your ability to stay calm. And it keeps you constantly on your toes, and you read things for tomorrow in case they pimp you. Some physicians do this just to break you down, while others are simply trying to help you learn and to find the end point of your knowledge, rather than as a put-down.

Such problems provoke in students an anxiety and drive to always be on top, even though, as one student expressed in dismay, "there is no way that you can win in that system. You will never be able to know all things, and therefore if you are asked something that you don't know, you can be seen as a dummy. And you are always going to make mistakes, and people are always going to react to you for doing so." The goal to always be on top can never be fully realized for exactly the same reason that all remaining work can never be finished.

The problem each student faces on a day-to-day basis is gauging "when enough is enough." For the first- and second-year medical student, practical resolution of the problem pivots around pacing oneself on the basis of structural indices—scheduled exams, classes, labs, and "breaks" provide definite benchmarks and goals students use to pace themselves. Toward the end of the second year, the schedule of exams, classes, and routines gives way to a pace based more on keeping abreast from day to day. Replacing a structured schedule are "floating indices" such as unscheduled events that develop in various classrooms, wards, and clinic settings, ongoing exchanges with faculty, patient interviews and write-ups, problem cases and emergencies, special meetings and seminars, schedules that vary between nights and days, and shuttles between clinics, hospitals, classrooms, labs, libraries, and home. A second-year student explained: "The first year, the objective was simply to anticipate and pass the tests. But the second year and beyond is different. Between working in the clinics, presenting cases, working up patients on one's own time, traveling, one has to keep day-to-day abreast of what's going on. You have to run wide open, seven days a week. There are no clear benchmarks as to when one has done enough."

The result is that the pace becomes based on the pace itself, which simply means a high level of activity and energy must be continuously maintained. Some students even rely on changes in bodily states and feelings as a measure of how much longer they can study, how many more hours they can devote to their clinical research. Upper-division students look back on the structured schedule of the first and second years as a "luxury," and bemoan their fate of having to now run "wide open" for indefinite periods of time. The progressive collapse of predictable schedules from the first through the fourth year of medical school and the accompanying uncertainty of when one is "on" or "off," feeds the drift in the student's life toward inundation. It generates a "natural" work orientation that strains toward a consumption of whatever private life may remain.

In addition to the high-demand workload and the problem of judging "when enough is enough," there are at least four other conditions that promote the inundation of the student's life by medical training. First, the study of medicine for many is an inherently fascinating and engrossing endeavor. It offers tremendous variation, drama, and wonderment. It can be extraordinarily challenging, and provides opportunities to channel one's humanistic and expressive sentiments into the service of saving or sustaining life.

Second, training for the practice of medicine is culturally and institutionally imbued with connotations of service, duty, professionalism, and mission. Many students even express a kind of obligation: since they were fortunate to be trained as physicians, they must provide service to those in need. Such sentiments include the common belief, particularly by minority students, that they should practice family medicine for the poor and disadvantaged in society.

Third, the practice of medicine is probably one of the most highly valued and rewarded professions in society. Being a medical student, and certainly being a physician, carries with it tremendous social prestige, status, and authority. Such profound reinforcement, along with the moral and ethical overtones attached to the work, all combine to impel the student toward a willing immersion in achieving his/her ultimate goal.

The unflagging commitment required of each student must be sustained for an indefinite period of time: four or five years of medical school, a year of internship, three to five years of residency, and then through an unspecifiable number of years establishing and garnering the necessary reputation to participate within a professional referral system (see Light, 1980; Coser, 1979). The commitment necessary to succeed in medical school is not viewed as a temporary commitment to medicine. It is seen as a commitment to be sustained throughout a physician's career.

### Impact of Professional Socialization on Family Life

Gaining admission to medical school is no small achievement. Not only does it represent a triumph and a consummation of many years of patient, arduous commitment and work but, as a milestone, it heralds the beginning of an entirely new status, identity, and occupation in the student's life. Among those accepted who are also spouses and parents, the event is typically regarded by the student's family as an equally momentous occasion. Attending medical school becomes a "master plan" for the family as a whole, a key to immense security, status, and success, and a chance to share in a highly honored tradition and purpose. The family looks upon accompanying the student to medical school as a potentially exciting adventure, an opportunity to live among and meet new families, and a chance to avoid the reputed routine, hang-ups, and "blahs" of a middle-class, nine-to-five existence. For these reasons the family response involves an enthusiastic commitment.

Once training begins, as inundation of the student's life gains momentum, its impact on family life is brought home by the student. Inundation of the student's life on one variable (occupational) generates complexity on all others. When "push comes to shove" and the need for "give" emerges over time, due to the demands of medical school coupled with the student's own commitment, the "give" must happen in the family and in private life. It does not happen on the part of the medical school nor within the student's relationship toward it. As discussed in chapter 2, students are severely limited, particularly during the classroom years, in their ability to fashion individual programs, schedules, courses, and pace. Taking course incompletes, dropping courses, and taking leaves of absence are only grudgingly granted in exceptional circumstances. The medical school's objective is to elicit maximum performance from each student.

Students' orientation toward medical training does not "naturally" drift in the direction of flexibility and individual accommodation. Students are very reluctant to approach faculty requesting special considerations for fear of spoiling their hard-won reputation as budding professionals. Many students interviewed indicated that on several occasions during training they had felt the need to seek psychiatric counseling, but had declined to obtain it from the available student health service for fear that word would get back to various faculty and spoil their reputation. Thus the family's initial commitment is put to the "acid test" by both the student and the medical school. Rather than remaining as an *option* for change in life, the commitment quickly becomes an unconditional requirement for the family to sustain itself. When the need for "give" emerges, it is within students' private and family lives that adjustments are made. The so-called test of the family's commitment pivots around its success over time in balancing its own needs, activities, and values in relation to the overriding priorities and imperatives claimed by both the medical school and the student. In the face of the student's inundation with the process of professional socialization, the family must engage in a complex process of balancing its own needs and activities around, within, and after the fact of the student's participation in medical training.

## Articulating Family Life in Medical School

As the intensity of medical training increases, a reciprocal tendency on the part of students is to control and minimize all competing demands and distractions (see Eagle and Smith, 1968; Bruhn and duPlessis, 1966). Single female students commonly express anxiety over whether they will ever be able to carve out the necessary time from their careers to bear children and raise a family. One female student, who was already married and had two children, said: "A lot of my friends think that I am really lucky to have a family and kids. Especially some of the female students, because almost all of them think that they want to have families, but they have absolutely no idea when they'll be able to fit such a thing into their lives."

For those students who are already spouses and parents, the tendency to minimize all competing demands creates a dilemma for the family. Any claims or demands the family may assert become increasingly vulnerable to being seen as obstacles and hindrances in the student's way. One of the many adjustments the family will make to defuse such potential conflict is to grant whatever degree of exemption from family life the student deems is necessary to live up to the standards of training. As Goode (1960:486) noted, an extreme option of exemption can involve the "elimination of role relationships," at least temporarily. The reasons for exemption are the same that bring about the inundation of the student's life—the unremitting workload ("because I have so much work to do"), the uncertainty and continuousness of the pace ("because I can't afford to take time off and still keep up"), or the high moral and professional values bestowed on becoming a doctor ("because this is the most important thing in my life to do now").[11]

The exemption the family affords the student is a *behavioral* exemption, not a symbolic one. As discussed in chapter 3, many students' involvement in medical school is symbolically seen as blended with or instrumental to their identities as spouses and parents. However, exemption can be interpreted as a symbolic breach of students' identities and roles as spouses and parents. The consequences for family life of seeing students' exemption as a symbolic breach are addressed in the last section of this chapter. The consequences for family life of behaviorally exempting students without seeing it as a neglect of family membership will now be examined.

Students' behavioral exemption manifests itself in two different dimensions of family life. The first is a physical exemption from family chores. Not only are students granted whatever time away from home that, in their judgment, is necessary for training; they are also granted a large measure of exemption from having to attend to such home-related activities as cleaning clothes, washing and vacuuming floors, making beds, cleaning bathrooms, taking out garbage, running errands, buying groceries, babysitting, shuttling children to and fro, and so on. Also, students are almost always exempt during the school year from having to work to provide family income.

The second dimension is a sociopsychological exemption. While in the presence of the family, students are exempt from having to be either expressly available, emotionally responsive, or engaged in spontaneous family activities. One student noted: "A lot of the time when I am able to be home, I simply don't have the physical energy to respond to my husband or children in the ways that I should. And this is almost directly proportional: the harder I am working at the hospital, the less energy I have for home." In the midst of "being together," it is typical to find students silently working away at a modest pace, sustaining an ongoing noninvolvement and disattention toward various family members and activities. Even on family outings it is not uncommon for students to drag along a book or two in the hope of taking advantage of a few precious moments on the road or elsewhere to review a dozen pages or memorize a few more facts. A characteristic boast of most medical students is their refined technique, developed over the years, of maintaining their concentration and studying in the midst of all kinds of distractions and disruptions. For the family, this involves issuing the student a special status allowing him or her to phase others in and out of immediate consciousness according to what the student deems most important. As Coombs (1971:143) reported, some spouses find it difficult to sustain the conditions for such sociopsychological exemption:

Although wives may enjoy having their husbands at home, it is difficult for them to remain silent, to suppress the constant temptation to interrupt. When they do interrupt, they tend to feel guilty. As one wife expressed it, "You've got to realize that he's a medical student and to leave him alone. You've got to put yourself in his position and to be consoled."

Although some students are patient with wives who interrupt and "want to play" when they should be studying, others become peevish and irritable. One wife described her situation like this: "He studies in the living room and I usually stay in the bedroom. When I walk back and forth from one room to another, he sees me out of the corner of his eye and it bothers him. I can't make any noise puttering around in the kitchen either." Other wives complain about having to lock themselves in such places as the bathroom and lament that they cannot talk on the telephone, play the television or radio, or open squeaky doors.

In addition to exemption, another important accommodative process the student and the family make to strike a balance is that of substitution. (Goode [1960] calls it "delegation.") Put simply, to the extent the student is exempt from attending to a number of family activities and needs, someone else must compensate by assuming additional responsibilities. Medical students and their families speak frequently of the various pressures and threats that impinge upon their situation. Included here are the problems of attending medical school, the family's problems of supporting and encouraging the student year after year in training, and keeping the family financially and emotionally afloat in the meantime.

Inundation of the student's life leads to a highly focused involvement with medicine. Such a specificity of involvement by the student necessitates a reciprocal diversification of involvement by remaining family members to meet those group needs which would otherwise go wanting. There is an "ebb and flow" in students' inundation with training, and there are periods of slack time and vacation when students resume more of the activities of spouses and parents. One student noted:

My situation keeps changing as frequently as I change clerkships. And each change involves a change in time and emotions and energy. This last clerkship in internal medicine, I needed my husband to be able to fill in all the gaps at home. *All* of the home responsibilities, etc. I couldn't do any of them. And he was real good about moving in and doing it. Other times I have more time and I say—"Honey, I know that you've got 'this' coming up, so I'll take care of 'this' for a while." So we go back and forth, trading off, trying to decide who needs what when. So it's an ongoing process.

During periods of inundation, students' spouses frequently express considerable concern over having to assume almost total responsibility for managing a family on a day-to-day basis: bringing in a partial income, cutting expenses and managing a tight budget, getting the student and the children to school, nursing illnesses, maintaining the home, doing the shopping and preparing the meals, and generally keeping everyone satisfied. As with the student, many times the entire burden for the spouse becomes too much, particularly when a number of problems converge at home such as illnesses, car troubles, money or childcare problems, pregnancies, and special occasions such as holidays. In such cases, because the student is neither in a position nor inclined to request special consideration at school, more distant family members, relatives, and even friends are called to fill in. During the four or five years of medical school it is not uncommon for families of medical students to seek "reinforcements" on many different occasions to keep the student in medical training and manage family problems.

When situations arise wherein specific needs, activities, and interests cannot be met, the family will typically "table" or reschedule such items until a later date. Attending medical school is looked upon as inherently involving considerable sacrifice. As Coombs' (1971:140) study revealed: "Almost without exception, wives expect medical school to be a difficult and trying time. They anticipate that their husbands will study constantly and have a total involvement in medical activities. Most wives (about 60%) found the first year of medical school to be about what they expected." When conflicts in schedules emerge between the student and the family, it is virtually taken for granted that many otherwise important things must be postponed until a more appropriate occasion.

The problem facing the family is scheduling its own plans and activities to conform to the student's schedule. If the student's schedule can be anticipated, the more likely the possibility of fitting the family back into the student's life. For instance, because the first two years of medical school are far more structured in terms of classes, exams, labs, the family is in a good position to schedule itself in anticipation of any upcoming breaks, pauses, or vacations the student can elect to use for purposes other than studying. As the training structure becomes less definite later on, and as students begin to think and behave increasingly like professionals, the training structure against which the family can schedule itself becomes more uncertain and irrelevant. Many family plans and activities tabled until later are threatened with being tabled indefinitely.

Implicit in all the adjustments the family must make is a vital assumption about time. As expressed by one student: "One of the things that makes it all worthwhile is that it soon will be over." Underlying the various accommodations the family will make in balancing its own needs and interests against the overriding priorities and demands of medical school is a set of definite expectations. First, an ultimate payoff is forthcoming, and second, there will be a cessation of the needs and priorities of medicine from routinely overriding those of the family. Both expectations are pervasively embraced by everyone involved. Both serve as a kind of buffer against the strain, workload, and sacrifices the family and student must shoulder. As time goes by, whether the family is willing to continue making the necessary adjustments is contingent on the extent to which both the ultimate payoff and the promise of cessation become closer realities or remain as elusive unfulfilled dreams.

*Balancing as a Way of Family Life*

A final requirement for the family, in addition to making the adjustments necessary to strike a balance, is to make those adjustments in ways which do not create even further problems. The family is expected to balance its own needs and activities in alignment with those of medicine in ways that are unburdensome. Both the student and the medical school expect the family to function in a kind of enduring, self-regulating equilibrium. The family is not supposed to be a source of additional problems; it is expected to be a "given" which can be more or less taken for granted. This is for at least two reasons, both of which are implicit in the above discussion.

First, if the family defaults for whatever reason in either exempting and substituting for the student or in tabling its own needs and activities into some kind of modest and convenient schedule, the student's situation—which already leans toward inundation—becomes unavoidably crisis ridden. For example, as explained by a student whose family was unsuccessful at exempting and filling in: "And I would come home feeling, wow! I'd really put in a hard day's work. And as far as my wife was concerned, I'd put in zero for her and the kids. And I just felt wronged. And when I was confronted with this attitude, I'd come home and the house would be a mess, and I thought, what the hell have you been doing, having coffee with the neighbors all day long!"

If the family does not take the necessary measures to strike a balance, the student's position ultimately becomes untenable. As a student's spouse explained: "If he wants medical school, fine, but help me also. And when I did say, 'I really need help, come home, I can't take it any more,' he'd come home and he was like, 'God damn, look what you're doing, you're sabotaging me, and you can't handle your part of the bargain!' "

The typical response on the part of most students when they find themselves straining to maintain some schedule or pace in medical school, yet confronted with unanticipated pressures at home, is to "bail out" of the family, at least temporarily. On a day-to-day basis, students take refuge by studying in the library, labs, classrooms, or friends' apartments. If necessary, they take private rooms in hotels or dormitories. Medical students go to extreme lengths, if necessary, to stay on top of medical school. (Mechanic [1962] found that Ph.D. candidates engage in similar defensive "modes of adaptation.") Exceptions to this tendency are very few. Thus, if the family is to maintain itself as a whole, it has no choice but to strike a balance; anything less will not work.

The family is expected to maintain itself as a "given" because the problems and pressures created by failing to do so generate havoc. The family must exempt, substitute, and minimize its claims on the student because its position in comparison to the extraordinarily prestigious work of becoming a physician is subordinate and inferior. The family is in no "position" to make any claims on the student which compete with those of the medical school because of its own social position; the institutionalized status and authority of the family is utterly secondary to that of medicine.

In contrast, the student's position is backed up by the entire tradition and institution of medicine, its honor, urgency, mystique, wealth, and power. Any family claims which contest or hinder the student's mission in medicine can be backed up only by whatever audacity and boldness the family is able to muster. But when "push comes to shove," the authority of the student's position inevitably overrides that of the family on a day-to-day basis, except possibly in matters of life and death. And yet the excuse, "matters of life and death," is precisely the ultimate institutionalized justification for the family's subservience to the position of the medical student.

For these reasons, both the medical school and the student expect the family to maintain itself in a kind of internally adjusting, self-sustaining equilibrium. Although this presents some very difficult problems involving exempting, substituting, and scheduling itself for the convenience of the student, the family goes to great lengths to comply. The family does so because it has to for the sake of order, and because such accommodations are socioculturally and institutionally expected of it. The family also complies because of the promise of eventual cessation of such problems and pressures, as well as an ultimate payoff. Although most families have some difficulty in specifying even an approximate date for the arrival of both events, their significance plays no small role in bracing the commitments of both family and student.

*Medical Students as Spouses and Parents*

The behavioral articulation of students' involvement in medical school with their identities as spouses and parents is achieved by virtue of the family exempting the student from engaging in many activities of family life, substituting for the student's absence, and scheduling its own needs, activities, and goals at the convenience of the student's schedule and needs. This is frequently done matter-of-factly and without many problems, except those of a practical nature (see Coombs, 1971).

Students' behavioral exemption from family life can come to be seen as incompatible with, or a breach of, their identities as spouses and parents, and then many problems of both a practical and sociopsychological nature can surface. In such instances, the symbolic grounds for the behavioral articulation of the student's involvement in medical school begin to dissolve, and engaging in the processes of exemption, substitution, and scheduling become primary issues of conflict and contention.

Particularly for female students, usually from the very beginning their student identity is not symbolically seen by either themselves or their husbands as "blended" with their identities as wives and mothers. Their identity as students is seen as neither simultaneously fulfilling nor instrumentally relating to, their identities as wives or mothers. One divorced student explained:

> As far as my husband thought, my roles as a spouse and a medical student were mutually exclusive. And I know that this is true of most women students because I've talked to some other women in my class who are still married, and it's been that. For women, it's all right to be good in your career, but you not only have to be good in your career, and you not only have to be a good wife, you have to be a superwife.

A single parent, female medical student echoed the same feeling:

> For a woman, you don't see being in medical school making you a good parent. When I look at it, I feel like I'm in medical school because of *me,* and that's selfish, because it takes away from being a good mother. I would never say that going to medical school is an integral part of being a parent. And in the same way that some women feel they have to be superwives if they are also going to be students, I feel I have to be a superparent. I mean, being a parent has to be separate from being a medical student, and I have to make up for this.

These testimonies support Epstein's (1970:90) observations:

> Most fundamentally, the woman professional must face a conflict in the hierarchy of status priorities in Western society. For women, the obligations attached to family statuses are first priority, while for men the role demands deriving from the occupational status ordinarily override all others. The

woman's duties as a mother override most other role obligations, her duties as a wife are second, and other status obligations are usually a poor third.

In the case of male students, their behavioral exemption from family life can also come to be seen as a problem, but usually for different reasons. Foremost is the problem of resentment by their wives. One wife said:

> I felt very jealous of school, and I felt like John was constantly choosing school over my health and well-being. I remember one time when John and the two kids were all down with a high fever and sore throat, and I had slept like five hours in a period of three or four days. I felt I just couldn't take it. It was too much! Then John recovered, and I felt I could now sit back and be taken care of—I needed sleep—I was exhausted. But John had already missed a couple days of the clerkship, and so he couldn't take the time off to let me sleep even one day! And I felt like, here I had been giving help for several weeks, can't you give me one day. So I called John at the hospital, and I told him that I just couldn't take it, I needed to get some sleep. And he said, "No, no, I can't leave." So I said, "OK, I cannot take it. If you don't come home, I'm going to take the kids and the car, and drive over a cliff!" And I was! So then he came home, and he was very angry and said that I was trying to sabotage his life.

Due to the feminist movement, many women are now demanding that all responsibilities of home life be shared equally, and that their rights to careers be given equal priority as their husbands' careers in medicine. One male student lamented: "I had all these demands at school, and I would come home and the only way that Mary would be willing to stay at home was if I would do more work at home. I felt that was totally impossible. I just had to get home and read and study, and she was demanding that I not do that, and that I help with the kids, and help with this, and I felt she was very unreasonable."

If individuals' identities as students come to be seen by themselves or their families as incompatible or in conflict with their identities as spouses and parents, there are a number of responses students will initiate to alleviate the problems. Yet due to the demand structure of medical school, each response introduces its own assortment of lingering difficulties. Students attempt to minimize the extent to which they require exemption from family life through two basic approaches. First, they decide to intentionally lower their academic standards and forego that extra level of involvement in research or studying which is necessary to get top academic marks. As one student noted:

> I know that if I hadn't had a family I probably could have been in the top 10 percent of my class. I've got the ability to do that, but I have other

priorities. I've hit a compromise. My academic standards are going to have to be a little bit lower so I can accommodate my family. And I've talked to other women who've said the same thing, that they are going to have to lower their academic standards, even though they've been used to getting A's. And I've learned not to let it bother me too much. But it has showed: I didn't do too well on most of my exams.

Another student noted:

> Because of my family and my involvement with my children, in comparison to other students I'm not able to read all the journals on the side, I don't know all differentials for all the different lab values—I just don't know as much as many students. I'll go in and present a patient, and be basically unprepared in terms of the pathophysiology. I mean, if someone is going to quiz me about it, I'm not going to have the answers. And I accept that. Part of that is that I'm not going to be able to put as much energy into preparing a patient presentation as somebody else.

Students will make an earnest attempt to equalize their participation in the family. As one student described: "Because both my wife and I have our own careers, everything about the house and taking care of our son is divided equally. Whoever is home first cooks, whoever has a few minutes runs and does the laundry. Of course, at times it creates friction, and sometimes we are both so busy that we get on each other's nerves." To prevent one's involvement in medical school from indefinitely postponing the opportunity to bear children and raise a family, some women even choose to become pregnant while in training and, of course, the wives of male students do likewise. This is a big decision, especially for female students, and also for men committed to sharing the day-to-day responsibilities of raising children. There is growing support, at least among students, for individuals venturesome enough to refuse to let their involvement in medical school flood out their private and family lives. As one student noted:

> Most women are really supportive of those students who become pregnant. Most of us were really excited for them, and wishing we could do it too, and wishing them the best of luck. I feel that the more people who are able to balance their motherhood and their studenthood, the better it looks for women. It's a big task. If X number of women in our class have gotten pregnant *and* gotten through school *and* maintained their marriages, then that's beautiful.

Unfortunately it usually does not turn out this way. By equalizing family life with training commitments and by lowering academic standards, students can attempt to minimize their exemption from family life. But doing so creates a number of weighty problems. First, in electing either of the two options, students open themselves up to the possibility of scathing criticism from the medical school as well as from other medical students. Medical training reeks of a "holier than thou" attitude and, as in some religious orders, there is a great display among members as to who is the most righteous, committed, and dedicated (see Damrell, 1977). Medicine is a most zealous profession and there is a great deal of put-down and mockery of the "old country doc" who is not up on the latest issues and developments and who does not display one hundred percent commitment to the mission of medicine. Those students who dare give equal priority to their families or who dare to be average in their performance as students, put themselves in the position of experiencing the "wrath of God." One third-year student described the reactions she received toward her being pregnant:

> You know, you have no commitment to medicine, you're not really interested in doing this, you're diverting your energy. That is what the people in my OB clerkship said. I got absolutely no support from them. And one person told me that I had better begin thinking real hard about having an abortion. And he said he didn't think that women should be in medicine, and that they were always going off and doing things like this.

Particularly in the screening of new students, and in the priorities and schedules dictated to students, the message is clear: there is no room in medicine for people with split loyalties and conflicts of interest, or who are mediocre or satisfied with being anything but the best.

A second problem, particularly for women, is the fear that if they do not prove themselves as available for training as men, women will again be discriminated against as in the past. Female students interviewed were aware that, statistically, female students historically have recorded higher dropout rates from medical schools than men (Lopate, 1968), and they were also aware that such statistics have had a detrimental effect on female applicants. Thus, maintaining an equal involvement in their families or bearing children while in medical training, intensifies these anxieties for women. The result is that in maintaining as active an involvement with their families as they feel they should, women generally think they must perform at an even higher level in training than other students. As they describe themselves, many women feel they must become superhuman beings—superwives, supermothers, and superstudents. One woman noted:

> So you find these people getting up at six in the morning to cook their husbands breakfast, and rushing home to cook dinner and spend time with

the kids, and then studying way into the night before they go to bed. So they try to be good as students, you know, 100 percent, and then they try to do the whole fantasy trip of being a housewife, too. They *have* to become superhuman beings. And you see women complaining about this.

The final problem students often experience in attempting to minimize their exemption from family life, which frequently requires them to lower their involvement in medical training, is that their lives become inundated on several levels at once. As Epstein (1970:98) explained:

> Abilities to deal with the complex roles of wife, mother, working woman, especially at the professional level, is still largely a matter of individual adaptation, compromise and personal arrangements, often characterized by strain. . . . The role strain experienced by the woman professional can easily become constant and enervating, aggravated by the ambiguity that makes necessary a new decision for each minor conflict, and by the often conflicting positions taken by other people in her role networks.

And because the student's position, by necessity, becomes a compromise between involvement in training and in family life, the possibility of not finding satisfaction or fulfillment in either area becomes much greater. One female student who felt great responsibility as a mother and wife, noted:

> When I'm involved in training, the house goes to hell, my husband complains that his needs are not being met, the kids complain. And the experience of tending to a lot of pressure at school, and then coming home and finding a lot of pressure there—I just feel like everywhere I turn, I am inadequate. I don't think anything has ever hit me as hard as that. But the thing is that you can't be a supermom and superstudent. I've tried, and I find myself failing at both.

Or, as expressed by the female student who decided to get pregnant during her third year in training:

> Well, as you know I'm now pregnant. And as a result of my being in school, I don't spend as much time "being" pregnant, and thinking about it as I had hoped to do. And I've been really angry that school seems to take so much time, and that I don't have time to get the baby's room together, or exercise as much as I would want to, and that I'm just really pressed for time. And I don't know what that is going to do when the kid arrives.

In summary, students initiate a number of responses to alleviate the problems that can result from having to exempt themselves from family life, from expecting the family to substitute for them, and adjust itself to the training schedule. While each of these responses partially resolves certain problems, due to the demand structure of medical training, each response creates another assortment of lingering difficulties. While students find they are able to achieve a behavioral articulation of their multiple lives, they are continuously plagued with problems of either a practical or symbolic nature. Medical students and their families soon discover that, no matter what ameliorative steps they take, they inevitably find themselves "damned if they do, and damned if they don't."

# 5.
# Private Lives and Professional Careers: Students' Management of the Future

## Time "On" and "Time Out"

Identities have relatively distinct temporal careers and individuals must grapple with the future in scheduling the expression of certain identities over others. In this sense, medical students are involved in a status passage which provides markers as to when one's student identity must take precedence over other identities. In completing the passage, graduation represents a date of possible payoff when the investment in becoming a physician can finally lead to the realization or support of other identities.

While students' private lives are inundated by training, the inundation is scheduled at times and thus predictable. Students are aware of which clerkships are noted for taking all their time and energy, and which are more reasonable. They are also aware of the recurring examination periods, such as midterms and finals, when one's absorption in training becomes all-consuming and maximal. Conversely, just as they can predict periods of inundation, students can also predict scheduled periods of slack time, vacations, and respites from training. During such periods it is typical to find students feverishly attempting to catch up and compensate for much in their lives that they have had to temporarily abandon, postpone, or neglect. As one student described:

> There have been times, particularly after finals, when I was just incredibly hyped, and I didn't come down for three days. I couldn't sit still. I didn't want to delay anything for anybody, I just had to do it. If there was a movie that I hadn't been able to see, then I wanted to go *now;* some friends I wanted to see, let's go. You always feel that there's a lot you want to do, a lot of experiences you want to take advantage of.

Students tend to use periods of slack time to think through and prepare themselves for future changes brought about by new schedules and clerkships, or to plan strategy about their future careers in medicine. As one student described:

One important use of slack time for my husband and I is preparing for the changes we envision are coming up and that we'll have to get adjusted to. When you are in the middle of a clerkship, it's hard to think about what you want to do next year, and it's important to take that free time and think about it overall. Who has time to worry about when you're going to have your kids and how it's going to work out? You've got this patient, and you have reading to get done. So vacations are a nice piece of time to do some thinking.

As important and useful as respites and vacations may be, in relation to the amount of time that students are "on," medical training provides very little "time out." Much of what students give up and postpone while in training cannot be recovered or compensated for on breaks. Thus all students look forward to the day of graduation since it holds a promise of cessation and ultimate payoff. While both the promise and the payoff are immensely reassuring in the heat of training, students commonly come to suspect that their vision of postgraduate life may be a mirage. Given the progressive collapse of a predictable schedule in the clerkship years and the demands associated with internship, residency, and establishing a professional practice, many of the conditions which lead to the inundation of private life in training appear to persist in each subsequent career stage. In fact, they may intensify.

Students note that the high-demand workload may be unaffected by the payoff of graduation. Internships and then residencies, which together last from four to six years, are notorious in this regard. Nolen's (1970) *The Making of a Surgeon,* and Light's (1980) and Coser's (1979) studies of psychiatric residencies, clearly document the continued "bust" in store for private life that a serious residency involves, particularly in managing an unremitting workload and a continuous high level of uncertainty and anxiety. A testimony by one intern, as recorded by Light (1980:50), indicated: "I knew I had to work hard, but I didn't know what hard was. I just had no idea. I kept thinking to myself, I know there's a routine here somewhere, and once I learn it, everything will be okay." Light (1980:51) cryptically added: "There is a routine, but not one the intern had in mind." In addition, Miller's (1970) study on the nature and impact of residency training offers even further corroboration. As Light (1980:50) summarized: "This work [residency], plus all the visiting rounds, consulting rounds, lectures, conferences and lab research and seminars, is simply overwhelming."

Similarly, establishing and sustaining a professional practice is more of a quantitative change from the rigors of training than a significant qualitative change. There are always more people in need, endless pregnancies, emergencies, and life-and-death situations to be faced, one more hour out of every day easily gobbled up in the fight against disease and misery. Although a nine-to-five schedule is now a routine which more physicians are reputedly able to enjoy, many do not, or they find themselves "on call" two or three times a week. In addition, students point out that in actual practice the pace varies according to a myriad uncertain situations and cases a physician must be prepared to handle. The work demands an acute mind, steady hands, patience, an eye for subtle discoveries and deductions, and plenty of nerve in dealing with calamity and risk. All this—the uncertainty, responsibility, and pace— yields a resolve, an anxiety, and a preoccupation to always stay "on top of it" and be continuously informed and prepared. Many students particularly emphasize the *responsibility* of medical practice. As one student put it: "While in medical school, the school makes the demands that are relatively unnegotiable, but the thing is that the patients take the place of the medical school after one has graduated." The intriguing feature of responsibility over life-and-death situations is that the responsibility itself becomes a positive motivating force that heightens students' involvement in medicine. As one fourth-year student explained:

> Responsibility becomes the great motivating force. And I'm just really getting used to it. When these patients come on the wards, I'm scared to death that they are going to die, unless I read about them and am really careful. And I've heard other people say those things, and for the first two years I didn't really feel that way. And the thing about this responsibility is that it is so much a positive kind of force, something that I morally want to respond to. And I feel like I am really digging down into the core of my insides or being. I think this is one of the reasons why a lot of people when they are interns just feel totally sucked in. But the suction is not negative, but positive. It feels good to be there.

Or, as a third-year student described it:

> This responsibility for your own patients and your own reading is much greater, and nobody is telling you to do this or that. You are learning because you need to have this information to help deal with your patients on a day-to-day basis. And this kind of responsibility greatly increases your involvement. I am thus much more motivated than I was before. When I was a first- and second-year student, I used to bitch a lot at having to put in so much time. And I'm putting so much more time in now and I'm not complaining about it. Except now I complain that I don't have enough time to deal with my patients. Now I would rather stay home on Saturday night and get reading done that I feel is important to me in terms of my patients.

Due to increased responsibility, uncertainty, and workload, many students envision that their future residency and practice are not easily containable and manageable. To contain such a career requires a definite set of skills which students emphatically indicate are not taught in medical school. Such skills must be developed in spite of medical training, on the basis of whatever *personal* ingenuity and resistance each future physician is able to garner (see Coser, 1974).

Many students note that, coupled with the unremitting workload, uncertainty, and risk, the physician's work continues to strain toward inundation simply because the work can be tremendously fascinating and intellectually absorbing, and the social and economic rewards are among the highest one can receive. In addition, the physician's professional oath and responsibility underlie a sworn commitment that is continuously evaluated by all other practicing physicians. Students come to envision that the so-called payoff after graduation does not relieve the conditions that bring about the inundation of their private life or significantly change their relationships with others in private life. The status quo prevails. This becomes particularly apparent in the private lives of students who are spouses and parents (by now the majority). As Coombs (1971:149) emphasized: "Graduation from medical school does not automatically usher in a 'golden day of marital bliss.' "

## The Payoff in Family Life

Given the prospect of continued inundation with medicine into the indefinite future, students and their families begin to foresee that, in many dimensions of private life, the problems and processes of family life in medical school are not affected by graduation. Certainly graduation from medical school, or at least completion of internship, more or less guarantees the family a change in socioeconomic circumstances. The family is accorded more respect and status; there is more money, more opportunities for providing an education for the children, owning a nice home in a good neighborhood, and for traveling and leisure activities.

However, in other significant dimensions of family life there is very little change. For instance the differential between the new physician's prestige, authority, and power, and that of the family, is greatly increased rather than diminished. After years of investing time and energy, the student emerges as an autonomous, revered, immensely skilled professional, who has been trained to act with a great sense of independence, authority, and confidence. In recognition of this, society grants physicians the license to carry out the work of medicine with substantial autonomy, including the right to evaluate their own professional performance (Freidson, 1970).

The family's position, particularly that of the spouse, does not undergo any fundamental change. After the years and energy invested in getting the student through school, internship, residency, and building a professional practice, the spouse's position becomes even more subordinate. This is particularly so since the only evidence of the latter's investment is in what the *student* ultimately becomes. The spouse does share a portion of the payoff that accrues, but this is an indirect enrichment of the family consisting of whatever side benefits the physician eventually brings home.

Inasmuch as the differential between the physician's position and the family continues to exist, the needs and activities of the latter will continue in the shadow of the overriding priorities of both the physician and the larger institution of medicine. As one physician's wife stated matter-of-factly: "Not only is his own leisure repeatedly interrupted by the telephone and the demands of his patients, reasonable or unreasonable, but his wife and children are inevitably forced to some extent into the mold of the life's work that he has chosen. . . . The home becomes an adjunct, to some degree, of the medical practice" (Howe, 1954:15).

As the need for "give" persists over time, it is still largely the family which will be required to exempt, substitute, and schedule its own needs and activities around the schedule and convenience of the physician. For example, the new physician will continue to be considerably pressured and/or inclined to claim substantial exemption from family work, thereby requiring reciprocal substitution by remaining family members. Coombs (1971:153) suggests that given the prestige of being a physician, sharing in the work of the family may be seen as a form of status deprivation: "Being accustomed to his privileged status in society, he may find it degrading to come home and be asked to take out the garbage or to perform other tasks which, in medical contexts, are defined as 'scut work.' " The payoff in no way structurally affects the expectation that the family function as a "given," an equilibrium expected to adjust automatically to overriding priorities claimed by the physician in the service of medicine.

For these reasons, while the student and the family may receive a payoff following graduation in terms of certain well-earned socioeconomic benefits, the conditions during training which required the family to accommodate the claims of both the student and the medical school will persist relatively indefinitely. The promise of cessation remains unkept, never forthcoming in many important ways. The necessity of balancing the needs and activities of the family at the convenience of the physician's practice of medicine becomes an end in itself, a way of family life.

## Grappling with the Future

Given the prospect of indefinite inundation by their careers in medicine, students, early in their training, begin considering a number of decisions bearing on the articulation of their professional lives with their future private lives. Students' perceptions of their future careers in medicine influence a number of decisions they must make while in training regarding their private lives. The process of considering the kind of medical career they want, with respect to private life, is a weighty business. One third-year student noted: "Thinking about the future is a major preoccupation. Sometimes when things get out of order in terms of things that I see happening to me, I get totally flipped out over it. I can't pursue my other activities until I resolve the major question. The decisions have so many ramifications that you can't mess up." Students' concerns regarding their future professional careers pivot around three major problems. The ways in which these problems are solved are overwhelmingly influenced by the attitudes, values, and goals students hold toward their private lives.

First, students must decide which specialty to pursue. This decision is influenced by the encouragement and recommendations of certain faculty members. On the basis of formal evaluations and informal kinds of reinforcement by the faculty, students are informed of those clerkships in which they demonstrated appreciable aptitude and promise. Such encouragement is part and parcel of the coaching and advising processes integral to the nature of professional socialization (Strauss, 1969). As Lyden et al. (1968:223) found:

> Students with higher class rank tend more to seek straight internships in major teaching hospitals, to be encouraged and recommended for these posts, to be sought after by hospital selection boards. . . . Conversely, students in the lowest class ranks tend to receive less encouragement and fewer recommendations, to seek rotating internships in nonteaching hospitals, and to be chosen for these posts (see also Kendall, 1971; Light, 1980).

Faculty coaching is complemented by the students' gradually realizing which clerkship areas they find most interesting and stimulating.

Above and beyond these considerations, students' decisions regarding areas of specialization are greatly influenced by their attitudes toward their private lives (see Skipper and Gliebe, 1977). With few exceptions students' selection of their specializations is a *compromise* between their future professional and private lives. As Lyden et al. (1968:213–14) found:

> Diversity [among medical students] reappears, however—and with a vengeance—when the student begins to make the critical decisions and choices regarding internships, residency, field of practice, type and length of training. These diverse patterns of decision and choice were the substrate of our investigation. Our data show that as career diversity reappears, personal and family background variables reappear as important correlates of this diversity.

As one third-year student explained: "Regarding a specialty, my choice is made almost entirely on its congruence with my lifestyle. For me it is very important to recognize that you have to compromise. You have to choose something that you're going to like, but also something that will fit your life goals; otherwise, you're going to get yourself into hot water—you're going to end up divorced or something." Or as another third-year student described:

> For instance, my private life has very much influenced my choice of specialty. I'm thinking about going into anesthesiology. One of the biggest reasons is that you can plan your private life, you can go to work at a certain time, and then come home and leave your work there. And you won't be bombarded at night with calls, or have to go out. But when I first went to medical school, I felt sure that I would go into family medicine, and from there I went to internal medicine. But both specialties are just impossible—you get home and eat, and then go back to the hospital, and there's just too much daily disruption of your private life.

Second, students must decide in which geographic area of the country or world to establish their professional practice. This decision is invariably based almost entirely on students' attitudes toward their private lives. Private considerations probably account more for the gross differential distribution of physicians throughout the United States than any other cluster of factors (see Jonas, 1978). Physicians' geographic preferences are not based on professional decisions concerning which areas are most in need of their services. As Jonas's (1978:68) study revealed, based on reviewing a number of published reports:

> Doctors are not at all evenly distributed. By county population size, the ratio varied from 40 per 100,000 in counties with fewer than 10,000 persons to 196 per 100,000 in metropolitan counties with between one and five million people. . . . A 1973 study of physician migration since World War

II showed that physicians tended to follow changes in the per capita income pattern, following the movement of higher per capita income groups.

Also, perhaps in keeping with the sense of independence and autonomy associated with becoming a professional, students' decisions on where to practice are importantly predicated on private considerations: personal attachment to particular cities and towns, proximity to relatives and friends, environments best suited for raising children, areas offering greatest prestige, economic rewards or opportunities (see Kesselman and Peterson, 1979).

Finally, students must decide how high in the profession they are willing to aspire. That is, given whatever opportunities are provided them, students must decide how much time, energy, and personal investment they are willing to devote to medicine. One fourth-year student observed:

> You have to make decisions as to how high in this profession you want to go. What kind of a doctor you want to be. You say, OK, I want to win a Nobel prize. Then, OK, you're going to have to put a lot of things on ice. On the other hand, if you want to be a family physician and work for Kaiser, then that isn't such a heavy commitment. For instance, and I could be wrong, but a lot of people who are not as compulsive as others are the ones that say that they want to go into family practice. But I know damn well that those people that just simply try to slide by know that they will not be the kind of physician to do heart surgery. And I think that a lot of people with this attitude and orientation to medical school are freed up to do a lot more outside things.

Another student noted, "If you're going to be a high-powered physician, surgeon, be in a good program and, absolutely, if you're going to be an academic physician, you're going to have to continue to give your medical situation highest priority."

Regardless of their claims avowed in medical school admissions, the vast majority of medical students are not interested in devoting the totality of their lives to the practice of medicine. What they look for, as in their selection of an area of specialization, is a compromise or tradeoff between their professional and private lives. Such a compromise is a difficult and uncertain matter when grappling with the future. Whatever decisions students make, there are still plenty of unknowns remaining. And the conditions that bring about the inundation of students' life with medical school persist in one way or another in all medical specialties— a demanding workload, medical uncertainty and risk, immense responsibility. Much as students may strive to carefully design their future professional lives, uncertainty and anxiety persist. As one third-year woman noted:

> When I get really panicky, and wonder whether my life is going to stay like this—you know, am I going to have so little time and always feel so pressured, and wonder how we are going to survive with having children. But then I realize that I am working about eighty hours a week. And when I think about establishing a practice that requires only forty hours a week, if that can be done, then so much more seems possible. And having a family seems possible.

Because students attempt to plan their future in the face of a number of uncertainties, as well as the threat of indefinite inundation with medicine, they hedge against those uncertainties with an increasing sense of adamancy: much in the future cannot be controlled by decisions made in the present, but regardless, students' determination to do so intensifies. There emerges a growing determination to plan one's professional future according to one's own bidding. As one student emphasized:

> Regarding my residency, I see these people that are really consumed by it, and I have to say that this is troubling to me, and I'm having second thoughts. Maybe I should look for another specialty where you really get to go home at six or seven. For instance, I think that I would like to practice medicine about thirty hours a week, where I would actually see patients, and then ten hours where I would be able to read and study. But whatever my residency will be, I *will* contain and control it. I'm just not yet sure how that will be done, or what the residency will be yet. But I plan on having some control over my life again.

And so, students' visions of the future feed back upon and influence many of the important decisions they must make in the present. Much that remains uncertain is managed by their sheer adamancy to change the future—a future, however, which refuses to relinquish a mirrored image of the present.

# 6.
# The Impact of Private Life
# on Medical Training

## Defining and Redefining the Training Situation

The overall training situation in medical school calls out and defines a specific identity: that of "student" during the first two years and "student-physician" during the clerkship years. The training situation also lays down conditions which demand a high order of consistency in students' behavior across time and space in the face of alternative situations. But students also participate in other situations and relationships, and they embrace many different identities despite their immersion in medical training. These multiple identities become mutually articulated and influence how students select their medical specialties and geographic areas.

Students' adjustments to the training situation are not in simple conformity to the requirements of medical school. Such adjustments are mediated by students' partially constructing the nature and significance of the medical school situation by drawing off of important aspects of their private lives. In other words, students' situational adjustment is a "role-taking" and "role-making" process (Turner, 1962; Becker, 1964). Becker et al.'s (1961) research revealed that the most important aspect of the medical school situation which students create is a sequence of perspectives on "how to make it" in medical training. Becker et al.'s research documented that, particularly during the first two years of training, students fashion a number of short-term and provisional perspectives that they use to orient themselves to only specific aspects of the medical training situation. They begin to concentrate on learning only what might be on examinations, rather than on "what the faculty wants us to know" or "all that there is to know." They fashion their behavior by selectively responding to what the training situation calls for. This entails the development of pragmatic and provisional criteria for what students consider important. The nature of students' adjustment is a response to a situation that is partly a product of their own making. Students' interjection of their own perspective into the training situation appreciably changes the nature of the situation in ways which a faculty and administration may find surprising and disconcerting (see Becker et al., 1961).

The perspectives Becker et al. (1961) documented extended from students' perception and definition of their situation in medical school on the basis of their specific identities as students. Their analysis, focused at the situational level, emphasized the specific identity of "student." The student identity and its accompanying perspective were treated as largely unrelated to and dissociated from all other identities individuals bring to training. In a small paper on "latent culture" published prior to *Boys in White*, Becker and Geer (1960) address the fact that students collectively embrace other important identities which derive from outside the medical situation, but which shape their situational adjustment to training. Thus there remain unexamined a number of other perspectives which accompany those identities and serve along with the "student perspective" to creatively make up and shape the training situation.

## The Multiplicity of the Medical Training Situation

Research on the medical school situation revealed a number of perspectives, derived from identities which students embrace outside of medical school, that complement the student perspective. While, as Becker et al. (1961) noted, the student perspective pivots around the central concern of "how to make it" in medical school in terms of managing an overwhelming workload, other perspectives students embrace orient them to completely different issues and result in different types of group activities and endeavors. For example, there is a distinct "Black perspective" based on ethnic identification among Black medical students. This involves an orientation toward illness that competes with the traditional medical model: rather than approaching disease as specific to individual patients, the Black perspective concentrates on diseases that result from social and institutional conditions such as racism, unemployment, and poverty, and that are common problems of a specific ethnic group. Students who share in the Black perspective are far less interested in esoteric and complex diseases which call for heavy use of advanced medical technology and specialized knowledge. They tend to be far more concerned about the common medical problems of hypertension, alcoholism, drug addiction, malnutrition, lead poisoning, sickle cell anemia—which affect Black communities in greater proportions than other racial and ethnic groups. The Black perspective is also more concerned with socioeconomic change and greater application of existing medical knowledge and services.

The Black perspective becomes expressed in the emergence of a number of Black student organizations, such as the Black Caucus and the Black Student Health Association. It presents a different approach to disease and uniquely orients students toward one another, inspiring camaraderie, Black pride, and Black responsibility. In addition to the Black perspective, there are a number of other perspectives, such as the "human potential perspective" and the "Chicano perspective," which have emerged within and shaped the medical school situation. Probably one of the most visible perspectives, based on political identities and interests of students in medicine, dentistry, nursing, and other allied health programs, is that associated with the Student Health Organization. As expressed by the Stanford SHO (as reported in Ehrenreich and Ehrenreich, 1970:245–46): "We are developing an increasingly large base of medical people who are understanding that the problems of community health are political problems, problems of power and control over the institutions which affect one's day-to-day life; that they are not simply the problems of applying new technologies to backward areas."

Beginning in 1966, various nationwide chapters of SHO based explicitly on students' identities as activitists and community members, stimulated the emergence of a number of innovative community projects quite different from those traditionally offered by conventional teaching hospitals and medical schools:

> Over ninety medical, nursing, dental, and social workers gathered in California to study and serve the poor of the state. In Watts, students conducted an audio-visual screening program for 4,000 children in the Headstart program. In the San Joaquin valley, students acted as patient advocates for migrant workers, bringing people to hospital clinics and demanding that they be seen without interminable waiting. Working with state and county health departments, students designed and executed surveys which exposed the poor health of ghetto residents. . . . The next year, in 1967, 260 health science students worked in three student health projects, in California, Chicago, and New York City. By 1968, projects had proliferated to nine cities with over 600 student participants (Ehrenreich and Ehrenreich, 1970:244).

A visit to any major medical school will reveal a number of other existing perspectives students have introduced into the training situation, based on identities outside of training.[12] Rather than attempt to catalog the various perspectives, an in-depth examination follows of one that has significantly shaped the medical training situation and that is derived from an identity which transcends the training situation itself.

## The Women's Health Perspective

Because women are being admitted to medical school in increasing proportions, it is not surprising to see a distinct women's health perspective orienting women to different orders of experience and interests in medical training.[13] All women do not necessarily approach medical training on the basis of the women's health perspective, and some may do so only partially. However, the women's health perspective has emerged within the training situation through students' mutual identification on the basis of their shared identity as women. As Becker et al. (1961:36) noted: "We see group perspectives as arising when people see themselves as being in the same boat and when they have an opportunity to interact with reference to their problems. Under those conditions, people share their concerns and their provisional answers to questions about the meaning of events and how one should respond to them."

Central about the women's health perspective is that it does not so much prepare women for "making it" in medical school in terms of managing an overwhelming workload, a high level of uncertainty, and so on; that orientation is provided by the perspective shared by all students. The women's health perspective contributes to the situation of medical training by orienting women to "make it" in medical school with a special concern for the issues, problems, and concerns of health care and medical training central to women. The more salient issues and problems of the women's health perspective are presented below, followed by an analysis of the impact it has made in shaping women's orientation to medical training.

Like most perspectives or ideologies associated with social and political movements, the women's health perspective is frequently polemical in style and biting in its criticism of certain groups and institutions. In presenting the perspective below, no attempt is made at critique, even though many issues are open to dispute. The objective is to take the role of the women's health movement, present the perspective as it has evolved, and delineate its impact on many female students in medical school, an impact derived from students' private lives and concerns.

The central issues of the women's health perspective pivot around four interrelated themes. The first is that historically women have been denied or have relinquished control over their bodily processes due to the "pathologizing" of those processes by the institution of medicine. As Ehrenreich and English (1978) analyzed, particularly at the turn of the century, the pervasive attitude of the medical profession toward women was that they were inherently "sick," and all natural bodily functions, particularly those related to reproduction, were authoritatively defined as illnesses. This included menstruation, pregnancy, childbirth, menopause, sexuality, and the overall physical constitution of women— women's bodies were seen as frail, weak, unstable, and vulnerable to, if not carriers of, disease. The result, it is alleged, is that the medical profession progressively became the seat of authority and responsibility over women's health care. Routine events such as bodily examinations, diagnoses, deliveries of babies, contraception, and so on were "medicalized" or became medical problems (Illich, 1976; Zola, 1972). The medical profession became the sole possessor of the skills and knowledge necessary to define women's illnesses in the first place, and to provide treatment and remedies for their care.

The second theme is that the historical tendency to define female physiology as pathology is the product of a pervasive, institutionalized set of sexist attitudes against women in society, and that those attitudes have been reflected by the profession of medicine. It is charged that the medical profession's orientation toward women's bodies as inherently "sick" is a cultural reflection of the imagery of women as being dependent, passive, emotional, intellectually inferior, and weak in relation to men. This orientation is seen as parallel to the ideology which justified the exclusion of women from the labor force, and which was used historically to deny women the right to vote, hold public office, or receive professional training. It is alleged that sexist images of women in medicine have provided the ideological basis for the exaggerated "doctor knows best" attitude, and the apparent condescension and arrogance of physicians who assume that women are incapable of understanding their own physiology and reproductive system, or who assume that most physical complaints by women are psychosomatic (see Boston Women's Health Book Collective, 1973).

Due to the alleged sexism embedded in the medical profession's orientation, many medical services are viewed as detrimental to the health of women in two major respects. First, it is asserted that the tendency to define women's complaints as psychosomatic has resulted in many real, organic problems being glossed over through the inappropriate prescription of psychoactive drugs. And medical definitions of women's physiology as pathology have resulted in a whole assortment of iatrogenic diseases (see Ehrenreich and English, 1978).

The third pivotal theme of the women's health perspective is that, since women's "illnesses" are in part a creation of sexist attitudes toward them, a new understanding of women's health problems is required. The women's health perspective specifically takes up a reexamination of the nature of women's illnesses, which has resulted in new attitudes toward contraception, menstruation, menopause, pregnancy, childbirth, surgery, drugs, and problems of sexuality and mental health (see Ruzek, 1975). The most significant conceptual advance has been the dissociation of women's physiology from imputations of sickness. Childbirth, in particular, a "problem" over which physicians have traditionally claimed complete authority, is increasingly being seen as a natural process which should be free of physicians' dominance. Women are striving to educate themselves in all aspects of the birth process—an education which physicians have routinely withheld from female patients. There is also a growing movement to take birthing out of the hands of the medical profession (see Arms, 1975). As Ruzek (1975:28) noted, many groups have "been advocating participation of women and their relatives in the childbirth experience, and questioning the routine use of anesthesia and episiotomy and separating mothers and babies." Others have advocated natural childbirth at home, reinstitutionalizing midwifery and using family members in assisting the birth process.

The women's health perspective casts a very critical eye toward the use of surgery and drugs to remedy many "problems." Individuals have documented the alarming number of needless hysterectomies and mastectomies that have been performed, and the negligence of physicians who symptomatically treat women's problems through the overuse of tranquilizers (see Chesler, 1972; Mendelsohn, 1979). The women's health perspective has also led to examinations of the extent to which women have been used as unwitting guinea pigs in medical experimentation, particularly involving relatively untested drugs, techniques, and contraceptive devices (see Wertz and Wertz, 1977; Illich, 1976). In general, the women's health perspective has provided women with a new and critical orientation toward their own health problems, a sense of responsibility to gain knowledge and control over both the facts and the medically perpetuated myths concerning those problems, and a militancy to demand an enlightened reform in the quality of medical services.

The final theme of the women's health perspective is that, for women to secure the rights and knowledge necessary to control their own bodies and selves, the problem of sexism in all major institutions, particularly medicine, must be eliminated. Accomplishing this goal requires a restructuring of major social institutions and particularly the emergence of a more enlightened and sensitive health care system (see Campbell, 1973). As noted, women are advocating an increased use of midwives in childbirth and resituating the birthing experience from hospitals to homes and other "natural" environments. Women have also collectively brought about the emergence of alternative women's clinics staffed by both professional and lay female personnel. The women's health perspective has oriented women toward creating self-help programs "where women learn to rely on themselves and each other for routine examinations and health care" (Ruzek, 1975:48).

There have been a number of changes brought about within the profession of medicine. Women have become critical of the nature of routine treatment. The purported condescension and mystique of the traditional physician-patient interaction is being increasingly challenged, and women have conceptualized problems such as "how to treat your doctor" (Blackman, 1972). Women and others have brought about changes in "informed consent" procedures, both in medical treatment and experimentation, and they now expect physicians to provide a clear and comprehensible explanation of proposed medical treatments and a summary of possible risks. The medical profession has been humbled by finding itself increasingly on the defensive in dealing with women. As Ruzek (1975) noted, the medical profession has had to come around to acknowledging many of the problems in medical care that women have revealed.

In terms of medical organizations, the women's health perspective and the women's liberation movement in general have served to increase the recruitment of women into the medical profession and allied medical fields. There is increased sensitivity to the need for greater numbers of female physicians who are more likely to represent women's interests, both in the politics of health care and in the delivery of medical services. However, as the Boston Women's Health Book Collective (1973:269) cautioned: "Lots of changes are coming, and women's clinics and health centers will probably be part of them, but for most of us for a long time doctors and hospitals as they are now will be part of our lives." The women's health perspective is as much concerned with the reorganization of medical services as with criticizing the present system. Many changes in medical services that have already emerged because of this perspective may be the beginning of a minor revolution in medical thought and practice in coming years.

*Impact of the Women's Health Perspective on Medical Training*

The women's health perspective has brought about the emergence of new forms of health clinics, new definitions of health and illness, new lifestyles, new areas of medical and social research, hundreds of articles and books, and much-needed reform in terms of women's rights to medical treatment, availability and quality of services, and the use of women in medical experimentation (see Ruzek, 1975; Olesen, 1976; Boston Women's Health Collective, 1973). The women's health perspective has also introduced salient changes in female students' orientation to medical training.

The reexamination of women's medical "problems" has generated a critical perspective by female students toward the way such problems are dealt with and presented in medical training. For instance, in matters such as pregnancy and childbirth, female students are now quicker to openly dispute and challenge the disease model when presented in traditional terms. Such occasions frequently occur during the classroom years of training. As one student noted, "some women that are big on home births have come down hard on professors who are too hospital-oriented, and these kinds of debates occur in the classroom all the time." In general, as one student noted:

> Women have brought women's issues into focus for medical students. At times when there were few women in medical school, issues of body image and images of women were not seriously called into question and reexamined by medical students. Women coming in have changed the attitudes toward obstetrics and gynecology, and they are starting to make a dent in how people treat female patients, and how to approach the female body and the female approach to things.

*All* the issues that have been called into question within the larger women's health perspective are now issues that female students feel confident to challenge faculty on; these issues are now fair game for debate, and female students know that the orthodox medical establishment must face up to the questions they raise and change itself in the process. In alerting women to the apparent inadequacies and misconceptions in orthodox medicine, the women's health perspective has revealed a connection between medical science and sexist ideology which pervades all political, economic, religious, and educational philosophies and institutions in Western civilization. As Ehrenreich and English (1973:5) noted:

> Medical science has been one of the most powerful sources of sexist ideology in our culture. Justifications for sexual discrimination—in education, in jobs, in public life—must ultimately rest on the one thing that differentiates women from men—their bodies. Theories of male superiority ultimately rest in biology. . . . Medicine's prime contribution to sexist ideology has been to prescribe women as sick, and as potentially sickening to men.

The women's health perspective has sensitized female students to the problem of medical misinformation regarding women's health problems, and the institutionalized sexism inherent in medical training, treatment procedures, and medical thought (see Campbell, 1973). Below, women describe their sensitivity to the problem of sexism in training and their vociferous reactions to it, as they find it operating against women as students and patients.

For women as patients, almost all students interviewed noted the tendency for women to react vehemently against sexist images of female patients conveyed in instructional presentations. As one female student expressed: "In the classroom years, women patients are almost always presented as 'crocks.' It used to be that whenever a patient would come in with symptoms that turned out to be emotional problems, those would always, always, always be women patients. But women now boo and hiss like hell in classes if a professor says or alludes to women inappropriately." Another woman said: "From my own experience, the way male physicians talk about female problems and female parts, the kind of joking that used to go on in anatomy about female breasts and vaginas, the slides that we've been shown to 'wake people up' in lectures— all that stuff of women as an object has had to change because women who are in the process of training are not going to stand for that."

Female students note that sexism toward them can be subtle. They also emphasize that whether obvious or subtle, being a woman is never a neutral attribute. As one woman explained: "I have been in clerkships where I have been the only woman, and sometimes I get congratulated for doing well in a bunch of men, and then I've been in other clerkships where all these men thought that I was just awful just because I was a woman. So being a woman is either an advantage or a disadvantage, but it is never really a neutral situation. You are always aware of its effect in one way or another."

One important example of overt sexism occurs when female students receive different training from that of male students. Lopate (1968:21) described the experience of a "woman who was the first graduate of a well-known medical school before World War I. . . . When she got into clinical medicine and the class had a patient with, for example, genitourinary diseases, she was asked to leave and go to the library for the period. Such restrictions were frequent at the time, but common sense has since triumphed over delicacy, and women medical students are now expected to learn the full curriculum."

Female students are now *expected* to learn the full curriculum, but even today the expectation may not be fully honored by the faculty in certain instances. One woman described a situation involving herself and three other female students:

> Usually you pair up in groups for some clerkships, and for several of mine it just happened that three of my friends who were all women made up the entire clerkship group. But the problem that came up in that situation

is that the doctors who were teaching us, the preceptors, were kind of overwhelmed by being faced with four women. So, for instance, we were never, never taught how to do rectal exams. We were supposed to be taught in surgery, and the surgeon was completely freaked out at the idea of taking four women in to see the patient and teaching them how to do a rectal exam. And so he said that we would learn that in general medicine. And we kept saying that this was clearly spelled out for surgery, and he just chose to ignore it. And so when we got to general, this guy said— "Well, you should have learned it in surgery." So they never did teach us how to do a rectal—it was just completely evaded by the faculty.

In contrast to overt sexism, female students note that subtle kinds of sexist actions toward them by faculty members are much more covert and difficult to challenge. As one female student described:

The ways in which sexist messages are conveyed are really subtle and insidious. Like, in a group of people, the men will tend to speak and address only the other men in the group. And when men speak up, the group seems much more interested. And then, when we get our student evaluations, there are certain things said like, they'll say that I'm "cheerful"— that's the kind of word they feel free to use for a woman, but you would *never* see that word used for a man. I have another friend, and her evaluation said that she was "well mannered"! *She had good manners and was polite!* These are the kinds of Pollyanna evaluations women frequently get.

Lopate (1968:16–17) noted that, up to and including most of the twentieth century, "the majority of women physicians have purposely tried to merge their identity and interests with those of the male segment of the profession." Due to the advent of the women's health perspective, women are opposed to the idea of "being made into men," and many now insist that their identity as women be regarded as equal to men. The battle against sexism is still being waged, both quietly and openly, and the position women are attempting to carve out for themselves gains ideological and substantive strength from the women's health perspective and the larger women's liberation movement.

Introduction of the women's health perspective into the training situation has strengthened women's orientation to protecting and enhancing their status as medical students. Women are now more prepared to openly repudiate sexist attitudes and actions toward them by faculty members, and they are more concerned about setting a high example in training to protect the opportunities for women to become professionals. Reciprocally, women are also very conscious of how far they should attempt to "bend the rules" to make medical training more accommodative of women's needs and values, without jeopardizing the status of other women by intimating that women cannot handle the present training situation. Women find themselves walking a thin line: the women's health perspective has strengthened women's attitudes toward themselves and has provided an ideological rationale for women to push for reform in medical training. Yet women do not want their advocacy to insinuate that reform is needed because women are unable to measure up to the rigors of present training policies.

On the one hand, there is a tendency to avoid pushing for any special considerations. As one student noted:

> There is a real strong pressure for women not to ask for special consideration. For instance, there have been a couple of times that I have been tempted to take a leave of absence, or even drop out of school, because the pressure was too much for me to take. But that carries a high price, because I would be damning a lot of women who would be the ones to suffer. When I was interviewed for admission, I was told that a lot of women have dropped out of medical school to have children, and thus I was going to be discriminated against because of that. So women generally, and particularly women with families, really have to make the same sacrifices as anybody else. We're not going to get any special consideration because we are women, or have families, or anything.

On the other hand, the women's health perspective inspires women, both individually and collectively, to push for "special circumstances" and general institutional reform. Yet both open them up to either the anxiety of undermining the position of women generally, or to the charge that women are not cut out for the rigors of medical training. As one third-year female student expressed, after she had made the decision to become pregnant while in medical training: "Having a baby isn't a wise thing to do while in training. When I was in OB clerkship, I really worked hard to make sure that I was doing everything else that people were doing. And at times I was really worried about how I might be spoiling the situation for other women."

Many women are not interested in simply bending a few unspoken rules or asking for special consideration in individual cases. The motivation inspired by the women's health perspective—to protect and enhance the status of female students—has given them reason to push for overall reform in training policies. For instance, Crawford's (1972:583) article in *The New Physician* sparked considerable controversy when she suggested that "getting young women into medicine is only the beginning. Once there they need programs responsive to their special needs or they will not stay." The overall recommendations Crawford advocated included:

1.  Reevaluating the need for a 75 to 90-hour work week while in training.
2.  Reduction of the overall time required for medical training.
3.  Opportunities for part- and half-time training programs.
4.  Internships with regularly scheduled hours, including part-time internships.
5.  New types of medical practices.
6.  Provisions for childcare services for female students and maternity leaves without penalties.

In conclusion, Crawford (1972:585) asserted: "It is a simple fact of life that women have babies and medical women are no different. Special provisions must be made for the woman who does not postpone childbearing until all her education and training have been completed. She should not be made to feel guilty about having a child during her training and should be allowed a reasonable time for maternity leave without penalty."

Recommendations such as Crawford's reflect many of the pivotal themes of the women's health perspective as it is applied to the medical training situation. They reflect the sense that women's needs must be reexamined in an attitude divorced from the traditional sexist mentality, and that women's issues are inherently legitimate and viable as grounds for restructuring training policies. Crawford is not suggesting that, due to some inferiority and inadequacy of women, training policies should be revamped. Rather, given that women are as capable as men, medical training must be reorganized to support students' identities and needs as women. Much as Crawford's recommendations were clearly based on the intention of strengthening and enhancing the status of women in medicine—a concern integral to the women's health perspective—those recommendations might be used by others as arguments why women may not be suited for medical training (see Daley's [1973] reply to Crawford).

While the women's health perspective orients women to a concern for enhancing the status of women as students, women are experiencing a dilemma over how that can be accomplished. Women attempt to fulfill that mandate by maintaining a high level of excellence in their performance as students within the *existing* structure of medical training. But whether they are protecting or undermining the position of women by campaigning for general reform in training based on women's needs, or in arranging training schedules to accommodate their personal desire to bear children and raise families—both options eminently justified by the women's health perspective—remains questionable and unresolved. However, women are optimistic. One third-year student, who was also a single parent, noted:

> I think as more and more women get into medical school, it is going to become more and more responsive to the needs of students generally. I think of the women students that I know that have kids. They don't do what the single students do in terms of putting in the hours. I know single men that would stay a whole week in a hospital and not go home one night. But when you have children, and you feel like you have a *right* to have children, then you say, "Look, I won't do that." Women who end up doing well in medicine *and* end up refusing to do those kinds of things, will demonstrate that things can be done differently. As far as clerkships go, women will, and are, making a big difference because they are unwilling to be pushed around as much.

The impact of the women's health perspective on women's orientation to training is revealed in the many formal and informal kinds of meetings, organizations, and caucuses women organize within the medical situation. As one student reported: "There has always been a women's caucus in my classes, particularly during the first two years. And they kept notes on things that bothered them more than anyone else. And these groups have been involved in protesting things outside of the medical school, such as rallies for a childcare center on campus, legislation regarding the suspension of monies for abortions, the Bakke decision, and others."

These meetings give women an opportunity to share their problems and bring women's issues into focus. Such meetings are frequently directly related to training: women speak of the several occasions when they have invited female residents to counsel them on what to expect on the wards, conferences with various deans to discuss policies toward women, planning strategies for various social and political campaigns both within and outside the university, and so on. The women's health perspective and the women's movement have cultivated in women a much greater appreciation and respect for the experience of camaraderie and the strength of being together. As one woman student described: "One morning I went to surgery and there were two women surgeons and I was the medical student. When we were scrubbing, these people talked about their children and their families, and they discussed just really human issues—we didn't talk about sports or the stock market, which is the general thing men talk about. And this was a much warmer and comfortable atmosphere for me."

Due to the women's health perspective, women have increasingly begun to see themselves as introducing an alternative to the traditional model of physician-patient interaction. To begin with, women claim that their orientation toward patients and illness is generally more humanized and personal than that of male students and physicians. As one student noted: "Women have also brought in a different emotional level. Women tend to be more expressive of their emotions. They cry and laugh more easily, and I think that these things have tended to humanize the process a little bit. Women are just a bit more open about their feelings toward things. There is less of this old traditional 'detached concern' and cold aloofness—being able to cry with the patient and empathize with the patient." One important indication of this is the greater tendency of women to react to dehumanized and degrading treatment accorded patients. As the former student continued to say: "Women have also booed and hissed to things that they viewed as being insensitive to patients. I think women have been much more vocal about that, just more sensitive to basic human treatment."

Women see themselves as more humanistically oriented toward the whole person, more sensitive about the quality of the relationship between physician and patient, and also much less aggressive in their overall demeanor. One woman commented that such a demeanor may even be rubbing off on male students: "Men are learning that nonaggressiveness has its place. I have a lot of women friends that are pretty low-keyed with their patients, and I think they are presenting a different model. A lot of men are into being showoffs, and they are very aggressive in letting the attending physician see how good they are being real flashy."

Whether in the future women will succeed in institutionalizing an alternative to the traditional physician-patient model remains to be seen. Many voices both inside and outside of medicine have called for more humanistic treatment, more gentleness and tenderness, more concern for the whole person, and more affective-expressive involvement. Women suggest that the advent of modern medicine, dominated by men, has brought with it a highly depersonalized attitude toward patients, with only minimal concern for the patient as a person. The advent of the women's health perspective brings with it a specifically humanized orientation, not only toward women, but toward patients in general. The introduction of this perspective into medical training has stimulated a heightened concern for a more humanistic regard for others. This is seen as appropriate to the way in which women should be treated as students, and the way patients should be treated as well.

## Identities, Situations, and Social Worlds

Specific situations may call out and define particular identities. Some situations, such as participation in medical school, tend to be highly demanding and specific in the identity they call forth in individuals. However, because students are participants in other important relationships, competing identities feed into and partially redefine the nature of the training situation. Articulation of multiple identities within specific situations leads to situations defining identities, and identities redefining situations.

Individuals' competing identities can create new situations. The medical school setting contains a variety of social worlds and "scenes" which medical students and other members of the university community create and participate in by virtue of other identities and common interests (see Strauss, 1978a; Unruh, 1979). Such situations constitute, as Strauss (1978a:122) explained, "universes of discourse" which pivot around particular activities: "The basic social processes of communication signify an enormous, unlimited and ceaseless proliferation of functioning groups, which are not necessarily clearly boundaried or tightly organized." Besides a "student culture" in medical school, there are a number of alternative cultures which become expressed in the form of many social worlds. The latter can be categorized into those making up an outdoor culture, an athletic culture, and a free-form intellectual culture.

The medical student community is populated by many individuals with interests in the outdoors, wilderness areas, and nature. This provides conditions within the medical school setting for the emergence of "outdoor exchanges." Such groups organize outdoor trips, provide rental equipment, and offer special classes in first aid and wilderness medicine. The activities organized by such exchanges reveal the variety of social worlds in which many medical students are involved. For instance, an "outdoor exchange" caters to those interested in rock climbing, surfing, rafting, skiing, hiking and mountain climbing, and snow camping.

In terms of an athletic culture, students participate in a number of social worlds of sport, and thus the medical school becomes a setting wherein many of those social worlds emerge. Medical students may play racquetball, squash, tennis, and basketball, be jogging and karate enthusiasts, or body builders. Groups and tournaments are organized, such as those held by the squash club, the track club, and the karate club. For some students, their commitment to a particular sport may run as deeply as their commitment to medical training, and their reputation as a basketball player, karate expert, or so on can be as important to them as being a medical student.

Students' identification with various social worlds provides the conditions for the emergence of a free-form intellectual culture which becomes expressed in a mini-university within the medical university. Classes, workshops, and conferences in different intellectual and substantive areas are organized. For instance, due to many students' identification with the "human potential movement," there is currently great interest in classes and workshops focused around such topics as "Developing and Experiencing the Whole Person," "Intensive Human Energies Workshops," "Women's Exercise and Body Awareness," "Yoga and Meditation," and "Shiatsu Massage and Eastern Medicine." In addition, there are classes in painting, stained glass, pottery, calligraphy, and tap dance.

While it would be a mistake to suggest that the social worlds and scenes found within a medical university are nearly as full-blown, diverse, or robust as one would find in a general university campus, it would be equally mistaken to dismiss them as irrelevant. Because students must continuously cope with the voracious demands of training, their free time and capacity to cultivate competing interests and talents are severely limited. But alternative cultures do emerge, and the reasons why they do are important to recognize. Social worlds within the medical school setting swirl and coalesce around different types of intellectual, athletic, and outdoor interests, giving rise to entirely new situations. Such worlds consist of universes of discourse and interaction. Students' view of themselves as diverse and multifaceted beings provides the conditions for the emergence of these social worlds, despite a training program which threatens to flood them out.

# 7.
# Conclusion

Sustaining a fulfilling private life is an immense problem for medical students. Medical training commonly undermines students' identity as adults, leading to feelings of infantilization, mortification, and dependency. The largely nonnegotiable demands and high anxieties of medical training tend to inundate their private lives and weaken their ability to honor competing relationships and commitments. Training also requires students to seek varying levels of exemption from their relationships with friends, spouses, and families, as well as requires others to substitute for them and schedule their lives into conformity with the training schedule. As involvement and intensity with medical training increases, students attempt to control and minimize all competing demands on their lives. If this tendency is interpreted by others as incompatible with, or a symbolic breach of, their mutual relationships, the symbolic grounds dissolve to strike a balance between private life and training; the processes of exemption, substitution, and scheduling become issues of conflict and contention. Such conflicts serve to compound students' feelings of guilt and inadequacy, leading to more intense problems of resentment, hostility from others, loss of moral and practical support, rejection, separation, and other failures in interpersonal relations.

Participation in medical school represents a status passage which provides markers as to when students' identity as students only must take almost complete precedence over other identities. But such markers also promise students a date of possible payoff when, having become physicians, they will be able to realize and support other identities and relationships. However, as training evolves, students begin to envision that, due to the intensity of their internship and residency, and the magnitude of the problems associated with establishing a practice, the inundation of their lives with medicine threatens to carry over indefinitely following graduation. All the above-mentioned cluster of problems issuing from the inundation of their private lives with training threatens to linger on, even intensify. In addition, much that students sacrifice while in training—the cultivation of other interests, talents, and relationships— begins in some cases to appear as permanent losses. After all, the years from premed through residency and early practice roughly constitute more than a decade of steady, near-total involvement—all of one's late youth and early adulthood. The question is not whether the ordeal was worth it, but how much of what was neglected, postponed, or abandoned can eventually be made up or recovered.

As all students ponder this in light of the payoff of graduation, with the prospects of continuing inundation of their private lives with internship, residency, and so on, they begin to hedge against such a predicament with increasing determination. Decisions students make during training concerning specialization, place of practice, and professional aspirations become overwhelmingly influenced by attitudes and goals they hold toward private life. However, the degree to which students are able to render their practice of medicine according to their own bidding remains problematic and uncertain. The prospect of a continuing inundation of private life strengthens their adamancy to prevent it from happening. In light of these findings, studying the impact of medical training on the private lives of medical students provides new meaning to much of what is commonly known about the postgraduate behavior of physicians: their behavior can now be seen in many ways as a compensation for, not an extension of, the medical school experience.

Medical training delivers a jarring blow to private life: a prolonged period in adult life of socioeconomic dependency and sacrifice, compromises in private relationships which evoke feelings of inadequacy, unfulfillment, and resentment, a system of motivation which thrives on anxiety, intimidation, competitive aggression, fear of failure, humiliation of self, and so on. The overall impact of professional socialization leads students to analyze, even before graduation, how they can structure their eventual practice to afford them a private life free of such problems and worth aspiring to. Possibly such an orientation is a consequence of all "punishment-centered" programs of socialization, as Moore (1970) described. During training, medical students work toward achieving compromises between their professional and private lives in terms of place of eventual practice, area of specialization, and professional aspirations.

The determination cultivated during medical school leads students to make many other important compromises which favor private matters in making future professional decisions. The strong emphasis physicians place on professional practice as a source of upward social mobility, pecuniary gain, and individual autonomy, culminating in an equally characteristic social and political conservatism, reflect further ways in which professional success is converted into private rewards. The postgraduate orientation of students is derived in part from having to ignore or neglect important developmental and sociopsychological aspects of their private lives while in training—a decade-plus struggle to overcome the tyranny of medical training and strike some kind of reasonable balance. In a culture which overwhelmingly cultivates private ambitions and incentives, professional compromises in the pursuit of private success could not help but strike physicians as being anything other than reasonable.

Much of this may suggest a profound cynicism on the part of students, evidence that the naive idealism which most brought to medical training was surely undermined and extinguished. Becker and Geer (1958:50) noted that "teachers of medicine sometimes rephrase the distinction between the clinical and pre-clinical years into one between the 'cynical' and 'pre-cynical' years." However, Becker and Geer went on to convincingly argue that the loss of such idealism only represents one of many situated and provisional adjustments students make in managing the demands of training, and that it is eventually regained as the date of graduation nears. While this may be true to an extent, my analysis strongly indicates that students' naive idealism is regained in a decidedly reformulated state following and because of training, significantly structured in favor of private life and personal success.

Viewed superficially, such an orientation on the part of students may suggest that the impact of medical training results in a significant compromise and dilution of their commitment to the higher ideals of medicine, but this observation obscures what actually happens. The training is meant, of course, to teach students clinical skills and knowledge, and to instill in them a commitment to high standards of medical care. Medical training intensely pursues these objectives. It is commonly thought that the training is also meant to instill in students a commitment to the higher ideals of placing the concerns of medical practice over private concerns, and that practice is an end in itself. Cultivating such an idealism in students is thought to ensure that the rewards of practice will not be based on private ambitions and goals, and that medicine will be as humanistic as it is scientific, practiced by persons with a primary devotion to the protection and enhancement of the public good. It is presumed that, by virtue of such an orientation, the semblances of a quasi-religious mission are rightly conveyed in medical training, as well as in graduation ceremonies when students swear by a famous oath to "Apollo the Healer" with all other gods and goddesses as witnesses. But I have found that medical training creates a strong bias toward private concerns.

It is thought that, because of their presumed orientation to the social good, physicians are granted the license and mandate to define and control the entire range of medical services available to the public. Moreover, the ways in which physicians administer these services are largely free from evaluation by that public. Such autonomy is not granted to physicians simply because they possess an expertise in matters which the general public does not, but because the training and high oath of medicine are thought to cultivate in physicians an orientation to utilize their expertise for the public good, uncompromised by private gain.

Yet students do not select geographic places of practice with a primary concern for those areas of the country which most need doctors, or specializations which are appropriate for providing basic medical care for the most needy (specialization itself probably does not serve this end). This may suggest that medical training results in a significant dilution and compromise of the higher ideals of medicine. My analysis indicates that while students' idealism is reformulated because of training, what seems to be a dilution and compromise in the higher ideals associated with medicine is in fact the professionalization of those ideals. It is the perspective of professionalism as it is operationalized in medical training which prompts students to structure their practice of medicine in ways which significantly favor private life and personal success. The operationalization of this perspective and its consequences are most clearly seen in the way medical education is structured and in the role models which faculty personify to students on how to practice medicine professionally.

### Influence of Professionalism on Medical Training

The structure of medical education inundates students for more than ten years, and in this time enormous sociopsychological and developmental deficits are created in students' private and family lives. Much of what students and their families give up or postpone while in training cannot be regained during the niches and breaks of training itself. The inundating features of training derive from the fact that the program is structured along strictly professional lines. The perspective of professionalism, as it is operationalized, leads medical faculty to conduct training as if it were a world unto itself, zealously concerned with no other priorities than the mission of medicine, oblivious to any competing priorities or concerns. It is professionalism operationalized which promotes the audacity of medical faculty to demand of students total immersion in training, and the relegation of their private and family lives to a secondary and tangential status to training: students are expected to give unequivocal assurances that personal matters will not hinder their total involvement in and commitment to training in any way. It is the influence of professionalism which leads to the exclusivity of focus permeating the relationship of medical schools toward their students.

During training, medical schools are not interested in dealing with any excuses, exceptions, or problem situations deriving from students' private lives. As Jonas (1978) and many others have indicated, it was the influence of the Flexner Report, published in 1910, which led to the sweeping infusion of professionalism into medical training, a perspective which gained momentum as medicine became increasingly self-protective and monopolistic as a discipline (see Freidson, 1970).[14]

Notwithstanding the ethos that professionals are a special breed totally committed to upholding and advancing the mission of their profession, the impact of medical training is so much at odds with private and family life that students become increasingly concerned with protecting it. Professionalism structures training such that it renders students' private lives irrelevant and to be held in abeyance. Doing so, week after week, year after year, heightens the needs, concerns, and priorities in students' private lives, which in turn leads them to begin structuring their eventual practice in favor of private life. The problem facing students is how to achieve a fulfilling sense of personhood, a mutually supportive private and family life. The adamancy cultivated in students to achieve this is made necessary by the untempered influence of professionalism which makes medical training a classic "greedy institution," as Coser (1974) would say.

The process of striking a reasonable balance between professional and private life is arduous, riddled with feelings of guilt, incompleteness, and unfulfillment. As quoted above, Dr. X noted that because a medical student is such a late arrival in the Game of Life, he or she attempts to strike a reasonable balance: "But by then he has given too many hostages. He is no longer that pure entity, a doctor. He has become an impure mixture of husband, father, colleague and doctor whose responsibilities to others, whose commitments and promises have begun to outweigh the pure considerations of the healing science." The lingering feelings of guilt and unfulfillment associated with being an "impure mixture" derive from the extreme exclusivity called for and morally demanded from the perspective of professionalism. The jarring blow of professional socialization sets up obstacles and threats to private life which lead to the inevitable sense of "comparative failure" in relation to "true" professionals because of the ethos of exclusivity contained in the perspective of that identity (see Glaser, 1964).

Regarding the ways in which faculty role models lead to the transformation of the higher ideals of medicine in favor of students' private lives, it first must be emphasized that the demeanor of faculty utterly personifies the perspective of a professional. For this reason, I would agree with Bosk (1979) that medical training, as conveyed by the example set by faculty, is foremost a training in ethical ideals as much as it is in clinical skills and medical science.[15] These ideals are contained in the perspective of professionalism, and they importantly circumscribe the higher ideals of medicine per se. The example set by faculty emphasizes the immense responsibilities physicians must fulfill in caring for their patients, the need to forever strive for the highest standards of care, to maintain the optimum in one's competence and skills as a healer, and to strive continually to protect the reputation and prestige of the profession. As they begin managing their own patients, students become very taken up with the responsibilities of their work, and this heightened sense of responsibility becomes a powerful motivating force in its own right. As Bosk (1979) found, students who appear to falter in upholding these important standards are harshly criticized by attending physicians and faculty, and their careers in medicine are made and broken accordingly.

The ideals which faculty model and pass on to students are significantly circumscribed within professional limits, and those limits do not reach and subsume the higher ideals of medicine. They do not include the ideals that one's medical practice should aspire to a primary devotion to society as a whole for the protection and enhancement of the public good, or to consider the health of entire communities as one's "patient" in a general sense. As Freidson (1970:153) observed, the commitment to ideals personified by medical faculty and practicioners is much more circumscribed: "There is only commitment to healing in the limited way the medical profession defines it. And commitment to serving mankind (or service orientation, as it is sometimes called) is limited to service in those ways the profession defines as being in the public interest." Freidson noted that professionalism, as it works itself out operationally, includes a concern for maintaining the prestige and position of the medical profession in the market place, a responsibility toward one's own clinical competence, and a responsibility toward one's own patients; it does not include a responsibility to society or the general public as a whole. The influence of professionalism, as it structures medical training and is personified by faculty, encourages students to go in one of two professional directions, or a combination of the two, both of which entail a circumscribed commitment to the higher ideals of medicine.

The first direction strongly encourages students to advance the science and techniques of medicine, which leads them in the direction of undergoing extensive specialization and ultimately becoming faculty themselves, as well as engaging in medical research. Students are encouraged to acquire advanced residencies in the most elite training institutions, under the tutelage of renowned specialists, and eventually to establish a practice affiliated with a teaching and research institution of equal prominence (see Bosk, 1979; Light, 1980). This direction is, of course, *the* most professionalized route students can pursue. To pursue such a distinguished career means that the payoff of graduation is never realized. Such a career requires that one's private and family life remain overwhelmingly subservient to the institution of medicine—one's practice, research, and teaching virtually become the sum total of one's life. As graduation nears, most students do not pursue this direction because they are not interested in devoting the totality of their lives to the practice of medicine; nor are they interested in having their work indefinitely flood out their private lives.

The second direction strongly encourages students to seek specialization and maintain a high level of clinical competence, and provide the highest level of medical care to one's patients. Except for the encouragement to affiliate with a prestigious teaching and research hospital (if one is "good" enough) and become sufficiently skilled to engage in those activities, the larger service ideals of medicine passed on to students are professionally circumscribed. Students are encouraged to provide high-level care to their patients, irrespective of who they are or from where they come, and to establish their practice wherever they choose. Such professional encouragement carries with it a circumscription of the higher service ideals of medicine because the mandate entails an impoverished service commitment to community and society as a whole. The mandate is made even weaker because of a cultivated commitment in students to maximize their professional autonomy in choosing both an area of specialization (preferably one that is professionally prestigious) and to establish a practice wherever they choose. Where students choose to practice determines the socioeconomic and ethnic parameters from which their patients will be drawn. A professional orientation therefore, max-imizes students' sense of independence and individualism in ways which strongly accommodate structuring their practice around personal success and private life.

In pursuing this direction, the highest combined rewards from both the medical profession and society go to those who seek further training in prestigious specialties, who work to provide the highest possible care for those patients who can afford to pay for it, and who strive to situate themselves in areas which provide the most desirable amenities for a fulfilling private and family life which a well-established practice can provide. There are no professional incentives to encourage students to do otherwise. The common derision by faculty of "old country docs," "general quacktitioners," and garden-variety community physicians re-peatedly suggests to students that those who settle for a general practice, who work in rural, isolated, or impoverished areas, or who provide the "nuts and bolts" of basic medical services are essentially losers, professionally speaking (see Bosk, 1979; Light, 1980). For those who do not choose to devote the totality of their lives to the advancement of medicine, the professional autonomy cultivated in them sufficiently circumscribes their idealism. The matters of where they choose to practice or what select patient population they draw upon to treat are, at the least, moot professional considerations or, at the most, important only to the extent that such decisions are sufficiently prudent to ensure that their practices are successful and maintain the high status and social prestige of the profession.

Due to the structure of medical training and the role models personified by medical faculty—all governed by the perspective of professionalism— medical students emerge with a commitment to ideals which have been professionalized. Such a transformation appreciably circumscribes the higher ideals of medicine—the service ideals—and cultivates in students, extending from deeply-felt needs, an orientation to structure their future practice of medicine in favor of private life and personal success. Such an orientation is an important shortcoming of the profession of medicine because it directly contributes to the maldistribution of physicians and the unavailability of inexpensive basic medical care (i.e., nonspecialized) for the most needy populations. In other words, the higher service ideals of medicine should not be considered as pie-in-the-sky dreams: it is only through their realization that the existing maldistribution of physicians and the spiraling costs of medical services can be, at least partially, overcome. Surely such goals are as important as these of advancing the knowledge base and sophistication of medicine, although perhaps not as professionally distinguished. Investment in their realization should be equal to the generous investments devoted to the professional advancement of medicine.

## Toward Socializing the Influence of Professionalism

It is essential that the question be faced of how the higher ideals of medicine can be introduced and cultivated in medical training. The obstacle is not the perspective of professionalism per se as it presently governs medical training; the professionalization of medicine has played an immense role in advancing the discipline and the healing art. But *more* professionalism is not the answer because, as we have seen, the perspective has its limitations and has brought medicine to the position it is in today. The dominance and exclusivity of professionalism in medicine needs to be enriched and socialized by a vigorous infusion of value-laden perspectives into the structure of training. Such a socialization would temper the largely unbridled influence of professionalism over the discipline, and broaden the philosophic ethos of training such that teaching the higher ideals of medicine would be institutionally legitimate and tied to practical options for medical careers and practices.

The perspectives at issue are not those associated with abstract intellectual traditions or other professional disciplines, such as sociological or psychological perspectives. Nor are they inter-disciplinary perspectives such as public health, epidemiology, or community medicine. All these disciplines are relevant to the practice of medicine, but their infusion into medicine would not bring about a socialization of the influence of professionalism or cultivate in students a commitment to the higher service ideals. The perspectives derive from the assortment of primary identities which constitute students' larger sense of personhood and which extend from their shared humanity as collective members of larger social groups, heritages, and cultures; i.e., the perspectives which accompany students' collective identities as members and heads of families, members of ethnic groups, residents of communities and neighborhoods, and so on. The socializing influence of these perspectives in overcoming the limitations of professionalism in medical training have already been felt, but their influence needs fuller recognition, promotion, and strengthening. Such perspectives stimulate a concern among students to structure their work and training more directly in line with the higher ideals of community service, conscience, and commitment. The most obvious example from the analysis is the influence of the women's health perspective within medical training.

The women's health perspective was introduced into medical training by virtue of students' collective identification with one another as women, wives, and mothers. It has cultivated in students a special concern for issues and problems of health care and medical training that are of central importance to women in general. It has generated a critical eye on the part of female students to the way women's health problems have been traditionally conceptualized and treated by physicians, and it has stimulated support for important changes in those conceptualizations. The perspective has cultivated support among students to root out instances and processes of sexism against women in medicine, whether they be students or patients. It has also led to numerous recommendations on how medical training programs can be reformed in ways which will attract more women to the profession and support them once they are there. It has resulted in the emergence of numerous women's groups and meetings which have served to strengthen collective solidarity and mutual support. The introduction of this perspective has stimulated a heightened humanistic regard for others, intended to redress problems of impersonalization and dehumanization characteristic of conventional medicine.

A number of other perspectives have been introduced within and shaped the medical training situation, all derived from collective identities students share with one another and with others outside of medicine: the Black perspective, the Chicano perspective, the student health perspective, and still others mentioned above. Such perspectives strengthen students' ties and commitments to larger social purposes, memberships, and communities as fledgling physicians. They thus contribute to the realization of the higher service ideals of medicine because they orient students toward structuring their practice with a heightened awareness of, and commitment to, community service and collective responsibilities. It is premature to suggest that such an orientation will also significantly influence students' decisions to specialize or not, and if so, in which preferred areas; or influence their choice of places to establish a practice. Certainly the perspective associated with the Student Health Organization of the late 1960s and early 1970s clearly encouraged students to make such decisions with a concern for reaching and treating the poor and the most disadvantaged segments of society. It also encouraged students to view their role as physicians as integral to their identities as community residents and leaders, thus tied to important responsibilities of promoting community activism and organization.

If the higher ideals of medicine are to be realized, the perspectives which derive from students' primary identities tied to family, community, ethnicity, and so on, must be supported and strengthened in medical training. To do so, educational structures need reforming in modest and reasonable ways, and a greater variety of faculty role models should be made available to students for institutional legitimation and support.

Reforms in the structure of medical training would include the implementation of proposals designed to minimize the gross inundation of students' family and community lives with training. There are no inherent reasons why medical training need be so much at odds with private life or deliver such a jarring blow. Greater flexibility in schedules could be implemented, workloads reduced, unnecessary course work and clinical grinds could be eliminated. Much of the tyranny and strain of medical training may serve an obsessive, ritualistic worship of professionalism, but the mountains of information thrown at students are mostly forgotten as they move on to new courses and clerkships (see Becker et al., 1961; Shapiro, 1978; Drake, 1978; Knight, 1973). Aside from becoming more flexible, programs could be made more practical. In addition to clinical clerkships, during which students gain important on-the-job training, community clerkships could also be designed in the service of practicing preventive medicine. Students could gain skills in working with communities in consciousness raising, education, organization. Training programs could be designed to support and strengthen students' identities tied to families, communities, and other institutions, and develop greater skills in actual practice and community service. As it stands, the voracious demands of medical training stemming from the influence of professionalism, obstruct the development of nearly all these types of skills and the knowledge necessary to use them. As Milton Mayer (in Harris, 1966:21) said somewhat facetiously:

> A doctor is, by definition, a man who does not have time. One of the things the average doctor does not have time to do is catch up with the things he didn't learn in school, and one of the things he didn't learn in school is the nature of human society, its purposes, its history, and its needs. . . . If medicine is necessarily a mystery to the average layman, nearly everything else is necessarily a mystery to the average physician.

To expand the breadth of such an orientation, training programs could also recruit more women and students from different socioeconomic and ethnic backgrounds—students whose commitments and concerns transcend the boundaries of upper-middle-class White males, who are sons of physicians.

Reforms in faculty role models could also be made along similar lines. Institutional rewards could be provided to faculty who are providing community services and who educate and organize communities to cope with health-related problems. This would require that the service component of faculty responsibilities be expanded beyond the perfunctory boundaries of serving on university committees and advisory boards or giving an occasional speech. Providing community service could be as highly rewarded as conducting research and publishing. Such reform would produce role models for students which personify the fact that, as physicians, they can and should also be, for example, active family members, community residents, educational leaders, and social activists.

If the higher ideals of medicine are to be realized, the exclusivity and disciplinary narrowness of the perspective of professionalism needs to be tempered and enriched. Such reform is possible through the infusion of competing perspectives into medical training extending from primary identities of students and faculty as members of families, ethnic heritages, communities, and neighborhoods. Such reform would socialize the influence of professionalism on medical training and practice, and increase the possibility that medical practice be structured by future physicians around commitments to priorities and concerns above self-serving private or professional interests.

# Notes

1. See Merton et al. (1957), Becker et al. (1961), Olesen and Whittaker (1968), Warkov and Zelan (1965), Coombs and Vincent (1971), Fredricks and Mundy (1976), Bucher and Stelling (1977), Mechanic (1962), Coombs (1978), Coser (1979), Light (1980).

2. A theoretical exception to the fractured images of persons contained within particularly structural-functional, systems, and behavioristic theories in sociology is symbolic interactionism. Interactionists have critiqued other sociological theories by drawing attention to this very issue (see Blumer, 1956; Bolton, 1963; Scott, 1970). They have attempted to "breathe more flesh" into images of persons even though, as Schutz (1964) convincingly argued, sociologists are inevitably doomed to the use of homunculi in analyzing human situations. All sociological theory and research must utilize hapless puppets, caricatures, models. No doubt, some homunculi are more imaginative and convincing than others, yet never lively enough. By emphasizing that individuals have *selves* and that, on the basis of ongoing communication and interaction, individuals continuously call out in themselves and in others multiple ways of acting and being, interactionists have portrayed an image of persons far more humanized and experientially congruent. Even in emphasizing the multiplicity of selves and the fact that individuals must continuously organize their multiple identities and involvements, interactionist studies of professional socialization have tended to restrict their focus to individuals as students only, and the ultimate product of socialization as that of a professional only. This is because interactionist theory and research focuses on episodic and situational levels of analysis. The promise of this is that by analytically bracketing their focus, interactionists have been able to examine the ways in which individuals build their lines of action together on the basis of communication and interpretation, rather than by explaining away interaction as determined by, or as an expression of, various external variables such as norms, roles, rules, and conventions. As such, interactionists have been adept at examining the processes through which individuals enter situations and proceed to mutually fashion their respective roles and "business at hand" through processes of interaction (see the classic examples of Goffman [1952] and Bigus [1972]). By exclusively focusing on how an interactant's identity and role emerge and become validated within specific episodes and situations, the identity of the individual tends to be seen as rather specific. The identity remains specific to the emergent definition of the situation. While interactionists may preface their analyses by emphasizing that individuals come to situations with an immense potential repertoire of identities and roles, the specific identity that eventually emerges within the situation is treated as unrelated to, and largely dissociated from, all other identities the individual brings to the situation.

3. In terms of the relevance of this admonition in identifying the goals and purposes of social programs, particularly for the purpose of evaluating them, see Broadhead (1980) and Deutscher (1976).
4. See Mendelsohn (1979) for an example of another medical heretic who came "out of the closet."
5. The following texts in qualitative methods were invaluable resources in guiding the collection and analysis of field data: Glaser and Strauss (1967), Schatzman and Strauss (1973), Glaser (1978), Lofland (1976), Johnson (1975), and Bogdan and Taylor (1975).
6. I am referring particularly to the dramaturgical and absurdist schools of sociology as conceived by Goffman (1959), Lyman and Scott (1970), and others. See Broadhead (1974) for further development of this criticism.
7. The only exception to this important rule involves the circumstances of minority applicants hoping to be considered under some type of affirmative action policy of a given school. In such cases, students are advised to reveal their minority status as an "extraneous" factor which may strengthen their acceptability into a "special" aggregate pool of initial applicants.
8. Although this study is based on an entire sample of applicants who were eventually accepted into medical training, almost all had received a rash of rejections from other schools.
9. For further analysis of the extrinsic aspects of commitments see Hrebiniak and Alutto (1972), Ritzer and Trice (1969), and Safilios-Rothschild (1971).
10. According to a nationwide study conducted by the U.S. Department of Health, Education, and Welfare (1974), the distribution of married students according to year in training was as follows: freshman, 35 percent; sophomore, 41 percent; junior, 51 percent; senior, 65 percent.
11. See Marks (1977) for further discussion of "scarcity accounts" as excuses and the function of overcommitment in producing scarcity in time and energy.
12. See Shapiro (1978) for a discussion of the apparent demise of the Student Health Organization.
13. As an orientation, the women's health perspective, as well as any other perspective, is potentially available to all students, and undoubtedly many students who do not share the identity that underlies a perspective are nevertheless sympathetic and supportive of the perspective itself.
14. Jonas's (1978:208) analysis of the voluminous *Flexner Report* discovered several recommendations for the curriculum of medical training to explicitly introduce students to the higher ideals of professionalism and to the social and preventive role of the medical profession in society: "Flexner described the importance of social medicine, that is, the role of medical practice in the social structure . . . [and] the inappropriateness of profit-making in either medical practice or medical education." Jonas states that these and many other recommendations were systematically ignored or deemphasized as the *Flexner Report* was incorporated into the reform of medical training programs.
15. In contrast to the claims of Barber et al. (1973), Gray (1975), and Crane (1975), who argue that medical training is virtually devoid of attention to ethical matters, Bosk's (1979:190) extensive research of a surgical residency led him to argue the opposite: "My claim is that postgraduate training of surgeons is above all things an ethical training. Subordinates are harshly disciplined when they violate the ethical standards of the discipline."

# References

Andelin, Helen B.
1963    *Fascinating Womanhood.* Santa Barbara, Calif.: Pacific.

Arms, Suzanne
1975    *Immaculate Deception: A New Look at Women and Childbirth in America.* Boston: Houghton Mifflin.

Barber, Bernard; Lally, John J.; Makarushka, Julia Loughlin; Sullivan, Daniel
1973    *Research on Human Subjects: Problems of Social Control in Medical Experimentation.* New York: Russell Sage.

Becker, Howard S.
1964    "Personal change in adult life," *Sociometry* 27 (March):40–53.

1968    "The self and adult socialization," in Edward Norbeck, Douglas Price-Williams, and William M. McCord (eds.). *The Study of Personality.* New York: Holt, Rinehart & Winston.

Becker, Howard S.; Geer, Blanche
1958    "The fate of idealism in medical school," *American Sociological Review* 23 (February):50–56.

1960    "Latent culture: a note on the theory of latent social roles," *Administrative Science Quarterly* 5 (September):304–13.

Becker, Howard S.; Geer, Blanche; Hughes, Everett C.
1968    *Making the Grade: The Academic Side of College Life.* New York: Wiley.

Becker, Howard S.; Geer, Blanche; Hughes, Everett C.; Strauss, Anselm L.
1961    *Boys in White: Student Culture in Medical School.* Chicago: University of Chicago Press.

Becker, Howard S.; Strauss, Anselm L.
1956    "Careers, personality and adult socialization," *American Journal of Sociology* 62 (November):253–63.

Berger, Peter L.; Luckman, Thomas
1967    *The Social Construction of Reality.* Garden City, N.Y.: Doubleday.

Best, William R.; Diekema, Anthony J.; Fisher, Lawrence A.; Smith, Nat E.
1971    "Multivariate predictors in selecting medical students," *Journal of Medical Education* 46 (January):42–50.

Bigus, Odis E.
1972    "The milkman and his customer: a cultivated relationship," *Urban Life and Culture* 1 (July):131–65.

Blackman, Rosemary
1972    "How to treat your doctor," *Vogue* (November 15):115–20.

Blumer, Herbert
   1956    "Sociological analysis and the variable," *American Sociological Review* 21 (December):683–90.
Bogdan, Robert; Taylor, Steven J.
   1975    *Introduction to Qualitative Research Methods: A Phenomenological Approach to the Social Sciences.* New York: Wiley.
Bolton, Charles D.
   1963    "Is sociology a behavioral science?" *Pacific Sociological Review* 6 (Spring):3–9.
Bosk, Charles L.
   1979    *Forgive and Remember: Managing Medical Failure.* Chicago: University of Chicago Press.
Boston Women's Health Book Collective
   1973    *Our Bodies, Our Selves.* New York: Simon & Schuster.
Broadhead, Robert S.
   1974    "Notes on the sociology of the absurd: an undersocialized conception of man," *Pacific Sociological Review* 17 (January):36–45
   1980    "Qualitative analysis in evaluation research: problems and promises of an interactionist approach," *Symbolic Interaction* 3 (Spring):23–40.
Broadhead, Robert S.; Rist, Ray C.
   1976    "Gatekeepers and the social control of social research," *Social Problems* 23 (February):325–36.
Bruhn, John G.; duPlessis, Andrea
   1966    "Wives of medical students: their attitudes and adjustments," *Journal of Medical Education* 41 (April):381–85.
Bucher, Rue; Stelling, Joan G.
   1977    *Becoming Professional.* Beverly Hills: Sage.
Campbell, Margaret A.
   1973    *Why Would a Girl Go into Medicine.* Old Westbury, N.Y.: Feminist Press.
Ceithaml, Joseph J.
   1968    "Appraising nonintellectual characteristics: the interview," in Douglas L. Lieberman (ed.), *Pre-Med: The Foundation of a Medical Career.* New York: McGraw-Hill.
Chesler, Phyllis
   1972    *Women and Madness.* New York: Avon.
Christe, Richard; Merton, Robert K.
   1958    "Procedures for the sociological study of the values climate of medical students," *Journal of Medical Education* 3 (pt. 2):125–53.
Coombs, Robert H.
   1971    "The medical marriage," in Robert H. Coombs and Clark E. Vincent (eds), *Psychosocial Aspects of Medical Training.* Springfield, Ill.: Thomas.
   1978    *Mastering Medicine.* New York: Free Press.

Coombs, Robert H.; Vincent, Clark E.
1971    *Psychosocial Aspects of Medical Training.* Springfield, Ill.: Thomas.
Cory, Donald Webster; Leroy, John P.
1963    *The Homosexual and His Society.* New York: Citadel.
Coser, Lewis
1974    *Greedy Institutions.* New York: Free Press.
Coser, Rose Laub
1979    *Training in Ambiguity: Learning through Doing in a Mental Hospital.* New York: Free Press.
Crane, Diana
1975    *The Sanctity of Social Life.* New York: Russell Sage.
Crawford, Carolyn S.
1972    "Today's women in medicine," *New Physician* 21 (October):580–85.
Daley, Timothy M.
1973    "Women in medicine: an exchange," *New Physician* 22 (September):548.
Damrell, Joseph
1977    *Seeking Spiritual Meaning: The World of Vedanta.* Beverly Hills: Sage.
Davis, Fred
1968    "Professional socialization as subjective experience: the process of doctrinal conversion among student nurses," in Howard S. Becker, Blanche Geer, David Reisman, and Robert S. Weiss (eds.), *Institutions and the Person.* Chicago: Aldine.
Davis, Fred; Olesen, Virginia
1963    "Initiation into a woman's profession: identity problems in the status transition of coed to student nurse," *Sociometry* 26 (March): 89–101.
Deutscher, Irwin
1976    "Toward avoiding the goal-trap in evaluation research," in Clark C. Apt (ed.), *The Evaluation of Social Programs.* Beverly Hills: Sage.
Douglas, Jack D.
1970    *Understanding Everyday Life.* Chicago: Aldine.
Drake, Donald
1978    *Medical School.* New York: Rawson.
Dr. X
1965    *Intern.* New York: Harper & Row.
Eagle, John R.; Smith, Burke M.
1968    "Stresses of the medical student wife," *Journal of Medical Education* 43 (July):840–45.
Ehrenreich, Barbara
1973    *Witches, Midwives and Nurses.* Old Westbury, N.Y.: Feminist Press.
Ehrenreich, Barbara; Ehrenreich, John
1970    *The American Health Empire: Power, Profits and Politics.* New York: Vintage.

Ehrenreich, Barbara; English, Deirdre
　　1973　　*Complaints and Disorders: The Sexual Politics of Sickness.* Old
　　　　　　Westbury, N.Y.: Feminist Press.
　　1978　　*For Her Own Good: 150 Years of the Experts' Advice to Women.*
　　　　　　Garden City, N.Y.: Anchor.
Emerson, Joan P.
　　1970　　"Behavior in private places: sustaining definitions of reality in
　　　　　　gynecological examinations," in Hans Peter Dreitzel (ed.), *Recent
　　　　　　Sociology,* no. 2. New York: Macmillan.
Epstein, Cynthia Fuchs
　　1971　　*Woman's Place.* Berkeley: University of California Press.
Eron, Leonard D.
　　1955　　"Effects of medical education on medical students," *Journal of
　　　　　　Medical Education* 30 (October):559–66.
Feldman, Saul D.
　　1979　　"Nested identities," in Norman K. Denzin (ed.), *Studies in Symbolic
　　　　　　Interaction,* vol. 2. Greenwich, Conn.: JAI.
Foote, Nelson N.
　　1951　　"Identification as the basis of a theory of motivation," *American
　　　　　　Sociological Review* 16 (February):14–21.
Fox, Renée C.
　　1957　　"Training for uncertainty," in Robert K. Merton, George G. Reader,
　　　　　　and Patricia L. Kendall (eds.), *The Student-Physician.* Cambridge,
　　　　　　Mass.: Harvard University Press.
Fredricks, Marcel A.; Mundy, Paul
　　1976　　*The Making of a Physician.* Chicago: Loyola University Press.
Freidson, Eliot
　　1970　　*Professional Dominance.* New York: Atherton.
Freidson, Eliot; Lorber, Judith
　　1972　　*Medical Men and Their Work.* Chicago: Aldine.
French, John R.P.; Caplan, Robert D.
　　1972　　"Organizational stress and individual strain," in A. Marrow (ed.),
　　　　　　*The Failure of Success.* New York: AMACOM.
Garfinkel, Harold
　　1960　　"The rational properties of scientific and common sense activities,"
　　　　　　*Behavioral Science* 5 (January):72–83.
　　1967　　*Studies in Ethnomethodology.* Englewood Cliffs, N.J.: Prentice-Hall.
Glaser, Barney G.
　　1964　　"Comparative failure in science," *Science* 143 (March):1012–14.
　　1978　　*Theoretical Sensitivity.* Mill Valley, Calif.: Sociology.
Glaser, Barney G.; Strauss, Anselm L.
　　1964　　"Awareness contexts and situated interaction," *American Sociolog-
　　　　　　ical Review* 29 (October):669–79.
　　1967　　*The Discovery of Grounded Theory.* Chicago: Aldine.
　　1971　　*Status Passages.* Chicago: Aldine.

Glazer, Myron
1972    *The Research Adventure: Problems and Promises of Fieldwork.* New York: Random House.
Goffman, Erving
1952    "On cooling the mark out," *Psychiatry* 15 (November):451–63.
1959    *The Presentation of Self in Everyday Life.* Garden City, N.Y.: Doubleday Anchor.
1963    *Stigma.* Englewood Cliffs, N.J.: Prentice-Hall.
1967    "Embarrassment and social organization," in Erving Goffman, *Interaction Ritual.* Garden City, N.Y.: Doubleday Anchor.
Goode, William J.
1960    "A theory of role strain," *American Sociological Review* 25 (August):483–96.
Gray, Bradford H.
1975    *Human Subjects in Medical Experimentation.* New York: Wiley,
Gross, Edward; Stone, Gregory P.
1964    "Embarrassment and the analysis of role requirements," *American Journal of Sociology* 70 (July):1–15.
Haas, Jack; Shaffir, William
1977    "The professionalization of medical students: developing competence and a cloak of competence," *Symbolic Interaction* 1 (Fall):71–78.
Harris, Richard
1966    *A Sacred Trust.* New York: New American Library.
Howe, Henry F.
1954    "Family and community relations," in Joseph Garland (ed.), *The Physician and His Practice.* Boston: Little, Brown.
Hrebiniak, Lawrence G.; Alutto, Joseph A.
1972    "Personal and role related factors in the development of organizational commitment," *Administrative Science Quarterly* 17 (December):555–73.
Hughes, Everett C.
1958    *Men and Their Work.* Glencoe, Ill.: Free Press.
Huntington, Mary Jean
1957    "The development of a professional self-image," in Robert K. Merton, George G. Reader, and Patricia L. Kendall (eds.), *The Student-Physician.* Cambridge, Mass.: Harvard University Press.
Illich, Ivan
1976    *Medical Nemesis: The Expropriation of Health.* New York: Pantheon.
Irwin, John
1977    *Scenes.* Beverly Hills: Sage.
Johnson, John M.
1975    *Doing Field Research.* New York: Free Press.
Jonas, Steven
1978    *Medical Mystery: The Training of Doctors in the United States.* New York: Norton.

Kendall, Patricia L.
    1971    "Medical specialization: trends and contributing factors," in Robert
            H. Coombs and Clark E. Vincent (eds.), *Psychosocial Aspects of
            Medical Training.* Springfield, Ill.: Thomas.
Kesselman, Judi; Peterson, Franklynn
    1979    "Why young physicians locate where they do," *Physician's Man-
            agement* 19 (October):92–94.
Kiev, Ari
    1968    *Magic, Faith and Medicine.* New York: Free Press.
Knight, J.A.
    1973    *Medical Student.* New York: Appleton-Century-Crofts.
Laing, R.D.
    1959    *The Divided Self.* Baltimore, Md.: Penguin.
Leif, Harold L.
    1971    "Personality characteristics of medical students," in Robert H.
            Coombs and Clark E. Vincent (eds.), *Psychosocial Aspects of Medical
            Training.* Springfield, Ill.: Thomas.
Lemert, Edwin M.
    1951    *Social Pathology.* New York: McGraw-Hill.
Levitt, L.P.
    1966    "The personality of the medical student," *Chicago Medical School
            Quarterly* 25 (4):201–14.
Light, Donald
    1980    *Becoming Psychiatrists.* New York: Norton.
Lofland, John
    1976    *Doing Social Life.* New York: Wiley.
Lopate, Carol
    1968    *Women in Medicine.* Baltimore, Md.: Johns Hopkins.
Lum, Carolyn
    1975    "The fascinating womanhood counter-movement: a theoretical for-
            mulation," paper presented at the Pacific Sociological Association
            meetings (March).
Lyman, Stanford M.; Scott, Marvin B.
    1970    *A Sociology of the Absurd.* New York: Appleton-Century-Crofts.
Lyden, Fremont J.; Geiger, H. Jack; Peterson, Osler L.
    1968    *The Training of Good Physicians: Critical Factors in Career Choices.*
            Cambridge, Mass.: Harvard University Press.
Marks, Stephen R.
    1977    "Multiple roles and role strain: some notes on human energy, time
            and commitment," *American Sociological Review* 42 (December):
            921–36.
McCue, Jack D.
    1982    "The effects of stress on physicians and their medical practice,"
            *New England Journal of Medicine* 306 (February):458–63.

Mechanic, David.
1962    *Students under Stress: A Study in the Social Psychology of Adaptation.*
        New York: Free Press of Glencoe.
Mendelsohn, Robert S.
1979    *Confessions of a Medical Heretic.* Chicago: Contemporary Books.
Merton, Robert K.; Reader, George G.; Kendall, Patricia
1957    *The Student-Physician.* Cambridge, Mass.: Harvard University
        Press.
Miller, Stephen J.
1970    *Prescription for Leadership: Training for the Medical Elite.* Chicago:
        Aldine.
Moore, Wilbert E.
1963    *Man, Time and Society.* New York: Wiley.
1970    *The Professions: Roles and Rules.* New York: Russell Sage.
Neugarten, Bernice L.; Moore, Joan W.; Lowe, John C.
1965    "Age norms, age constraints and adult socialization," *American
        Journal of Sociology* 70 (May):710–17.
Nolen, William
1970    *The Making of a Surgeon.* New York: Random House.
Olesen, Virginia
1976    *Women and Their Health.* Washington, D.C.: U.S. Department of
        Health, Education, and Welfare, National Technical Information
        Service.
Olesen, Virginia; Whittaker, Elvi W.
1968    *The Silent Dialogue: A Study in the Social Psychology of Professional
        Socialization.* San Francisco: Jossey-Bass.
Parsons, Talcott
1951    *The Social System.* Glencoe, Ill.: Free Press.
Pennell, Marryland; Slowell, Shirlene
1975    *Women in Health Careers.* Washington, D.C.: American Public
        Health Association.
Ritzer, George; Trice, Harrison M.
1969    "An empirical study of Howard Becker's side-bet theory," *Social
        Forces* 47 (June):475–78.
Rosenberg, Mark L.
1973    "Increasing the efficiency of medical school admissions," *Journal
        of Medical Education* 48 (August):707–17.
Rosow, Irving; Rose, K. Daniel
1972    "Divorce among doctors," *Journal of Marriage and the Family* 34
        (November):587–98.
Ruzek, Sheryl K.
1975    *Women and Health Care.* Evanston, Ill.: Northwestern University
        Program on Women.
Safilios-Rothschild, Constantina
1971    "Towards the conceptualization of work commitment," *Human
        Relations* 24 (December):489–93.

Schatzman, Leonard; Strauss, Anselm L.
1966     "A sociology of psychiatry: a perspective and organizing foci,"
         *Social Problems* 14 (Summer):3–17.
1973     *Field Research: Strategies for a Natural Sociology.* Englewood Cliffs,
         N.J.: Prentice-Hall.

Schutz, Alfred
1964     *Collected Papers: Studies in Social Theory.* The Hague: Martinus
         Nijhoff.
1967     *Collected Papers: The Problem of Social Reality.* The Hague: Mar-
         tinus Nijhoff.

Scott, Marvin B.
1970     "Functional analysis: a statement of problems," in Gregory P. Stone
         and Harvey A. Farberman (eds.), *Social Psychology through Symbolic
         Interaction.* Waltham, Mass.: Xerox College.

Shapiro, Martin
1978     *Getting Doctored: Critical Reflections on Becoming a Physician.*
         Kitchener, Ontario: Between the Lines.

Shibutani, Tamotsu
1955     "Reference groups as perspectives," *American Journal of Sociology*
         60 (January):562–69.

Skipper, James K.; Gliebe, Werner A.
1977     "Forgotten persons: physicians' wives and their influence on medical
         career decisions," *Journal of Medical Education* 52 (Septem-
         ber):764–66.

Stone, Gregory P.
1962     "Appearance and the self," in Arnold Rose (ed.), *Human Behavior
         and Social Processes.* Boston: Houghton Mifflin.

Stone, Gregory P.; Farberman, Harvey A.
1970     *Social Psychology through Symbolic Interaction.* Waltham, Mass.:
         Xerox College.

Strauss, Anselm L.
1969     *Mirrors and Masks.* San Francisco: Sociology.
1978     *Negotiations: Varieties, Contexts, Processes and Social Order.* San
         Francisco: Jossey-Bass.
1978a    "A social world perspective," in Norman K. Denzin (ed.), *Studies
         in Symbolic Interaction,* vol. 1. Greenwich, Conn.: JAI.

Travisano, Richard V.
1970     "Alternation and conversion as qualitatively different transfor-
         mations," in Gregory P. Stone and Harvey A. Farberman (eds.),
         *Social Psychology through Symbolic Interaction.* Waltham, Mass.:
         Xerox College.

Tringo, John L.
1970     "The hierarchy of preference toward disability groups," *Journal of
         Special Education* 4 (Summer):295–306.

Truman, Stanley R.
1951     *The Doctor: His Career, His Business, His Human Relations.*
         Baltimore, Md.: Williams & Wilkins.
Turner, Ralph
1962     "Role-making: process versus conformity," in Arnold Rose (ed.),
         *Human Behavior and Social Processes.* Boston: Houghton Mifflin.
U.S. Department of Health, Education, and Welfare
1974     *How Medical Students Finance Their Education.* Washington, D.C.:
         Government Printing Office.
Unruh, David R.
1979     "Characteristics and types of participation in social worlds," *Symbolic Interaction* 2 (Fall):115–29.
Warkov, Seymour; Zelan, Joseph
1965     *Lawyers in the Making.* Chicago: Aldine.
Wertz, Richard W.; Wertz, Dorothy C.
1977     *Lying-In: A History of Childbirth in America.* New York: Schocken.
Whyte, William Foote
1943     *Street Corner Society.* Chicago: University of Chicago Press.
Zabarenko, Ralph N.; Zabarenko, Lucy M.
1978     *The Doctor Tree: Developmental Stages in the Growth of Physicians.*
         Pittsburgh, Penn.: University of Pittsburgh Press.
Zola, Irving
1972     "Medicine as an institution of social control," *The Sociological Review* 20 (November):487–504.

# Index

Adult development: age-norms, 53; alternation, 36–37; ambiguous stages, 53–54; conversion, 36–37; situated adjustments, 35
Alutto, Joseph A., 114
Andelin, Helen B., 39
Application to medical school: rejection causes, 25–27; discrimination, 24; facework, 18–27; foreshadowed problems in training, 15–18, 27–33; the interview, 21–27; meaning of, 62–63; the "pitch," 15–16, 22; preparing for, 20–21
Arms, Suzanne, 90
Articulation of identities, concept of, 10–11

Barber, Bernard, 114
Becker, Howard S., 11, 17, 35, 45, 59, 60, 85–86, 88, 103, 110, 113
Berger, Peter L., 51
Best, William R., 58
Bigus, Odis E., 113
Blackman, Rosemary, 91
Black medical students, 86–87
Blumer, Herbert, 11, 113
Bogdan, Robert, 114
Bolton, Charles D., 113
Bosk, Charles L., 105–108, 114
Boston Women's Health Book Collective, 89, 91
Broadhead, Robert S., 5, 114
Bruhn, John G., 63
Bucher, Rue, 113

Campbell, Margaret A., 48, 90, 92
Caplan, Robert D., 57
Ceithaml, Joseph J., 16, 23
Chesler, Phyllis, 90
Children, choosing career over, 51–52
Christe, Richard, 45

Coombs, Robert H., 4, 64, 66, 69, 78–79, 113
Cory, Donald Webster, 19
Coser, Lewis, 58, 78, 105
Coser, Rose Laub, 60, 62, 76, 113
Crane, Diana, 114
Crawford, Carolyn S., 95–96

Daley, Timothy M., 96
Damrell, Joseph, 72
Davis, Fred, 4, 37
Deutscher, Irwin, 114
Divorce. See physicians
Douglas, Jack D., 2
Drake, Donald, 17, 19, 110
Dr. X, ix–x, 5, 53
duPlessis, Andrea, 63

Eagle, John R., 63
Ehrenreich, Barbara, 42, 87–89, 92
Ehrenreich, John, 87
English, Deirdre, 88–89, 92
Emerson, Joan P., 30
Epstein, Cynthia Fuchs, 39, 43–44, 69, 73
Eron, Leonard D., 45, 59
Everyday life, study of, 2

Facework; anticipatory identification, 20; categorical identification, 20–21; concept of, 13–18; individuation, 21–25; normalization, 25–27
Faculty: attitudes toward student families, 16, 27, 62, 67–68, 79; attitudes toward training, 16–17, 72; elitism of, 72, 106–108; as role models, 105–108
Families: expectations of training, 63; as "givens," 67; position in training, 68–79

Family life: adjustments to training, 63–67, 70–74; balancing demands, 67–68; delegation of responsibilities, 65–66; payoff of training, 78–80; problems in training, 62–68, 101–102; students' exemption from, 63–65, 69–70; student participation in, 71–74
Farberman, Harvey A., 52
Feldman, Saul D., 4, 18
Foote, Nelson N., 38
Flexner Report, 105, 114
Fox, Renée C., 29, 60
Fredricks, Marcel A., 4, 36, 113
Freidson, Eliot, 28, 79, 105–106
French, John R.P., 57

Garfinkel, Harold, 2, 41
Geer, Blanche, 45, 59, 86, 103
Glaser, Barney G., 2, 8–10, 12, 19, 55, 105, 114
Glazer, Myron, 6
Gliebe, Werner A., 80
Goffman, Erving, 15, 18–19, 23, 113–114
Goode, William J., 63, 65
Gray Bradford H., 114
Gross, Edward, 19

Haas, Jack, 29
Harris, Richard, 111
Howe, Henry F., 79
Hrebiniak, Lawrence G., 114
Hughes, Everett C., 37
Huntington, Mary Jean, 36

Identification, concept of, 38
Identity: components of, 38–41; definition of, 38; devalued, 39; impure mixtures, ix, 105; social value of, 39
Illich, Ivan, 89–90
Impression management, conveying competence, 29–30. See also Facework
Inundation, concept of, 10, 57–59
Irwin, John, 38

Johnson, John M., 114
Jonas, Steven, 81, 105, 114

Kendall, Patricia L., 80
Kesselman, Judi, 82

Kiev, Ari, 42
Knight, J.A., 36, 110

Laing, R.D., 41
Leif, Harold L., 58
Lemert, Edwin M., 58
Leroy, John P., 19
Levitt, L.P., 58
Light, Donald, 29, 62, 76, 80, 107–108, 113
Lofland, John, 114
Lopate, Carol, 24, 26, 48, 51, 72, 93–94
Lorber, Judith, 28
Luckman, Thomas, 51
Lum, Carolyn, 39
Lyden, Fremont J., 80–81
Lyman, Stanford M., 114

Marks, Stephen R., 18, 31, 57, 114
Mayer, Milton, 111
McCue, Jack D., x
Mechanic, David, 68, 113
Medical careers, 12
Medical faculty. See Faculty
Medical schools: attitudes toward training, 16–17; as greedy institutions, 58, 105; priorities, 16–17. See also Training situation
Medical settings, diversity of, 98–100
Medical students: as adults, 53–55; cloak of competence, 29; claim of professionalism, 27–29; compulsiveness, 58–59; cynicism of, 103; deciding place of practice, 81–82; deciding area of specialization, 80–81; dropouts, 72; as fathers, 43–44; as husbands, 43–44; as men, 42–43; orientation to training, 17, 62–63; problems of embarrassment, 28–30; professional demeanor of, 28–30; professional identity of, 27, 30, 36; pregnant, 71–73; resources of, 57–58; as single parents, 69; as spouses and parents, 68–74; training goals, 43–46, 82; visions of the future, 78, 80–83; as women, 41–42, 47–52. See also Women medical students
Medical training: as alibi, 55; characteristics of, 59–62; doctrinal conversion, 39; as an excuse, 63; family's

position in, 68–69, 79; impact on private life, 101; impact of Women's Health Perspective, 91–98; infantilizing effects, 54–55; influence of professionalism, 104–108; masculinizing effects, 48–49; payoff of, 66–67, 78–80; pace of, 60–61; "pimping," 28, 60; reforms, 95–96, 110–111; schedule of, 75–76; social value of, 49; as status passage to adulthood, 53–55; stigmatizing effects of, 49–50; uncertainty in, 60; workload, 59–60. *See also* Application to medical school

Mendelsohn, Robert S., 90, 114

Merton, Robert K., 17, 45, 113

Miller, Stephen J., 76

Moore, Wilbert E., 14, 57, 102

Multiple identities: behavioral articulation of, 57; compartmentalization of, 40–41; disclosure of, 19, 22–23; forms of symbolic calculi, 41–47; ranking of, 39–42; symbolic articulation of, 4, 38–41; temporal articulation of, 75–78

Mundy, Paul, 4, 36, 113

Neugarten, Bernice L., 53

Nolen, William, 76

Olesen, Virginia, 3–5, 91, 113

Parsons, Talcott, 32

Participant observation: gaining entree, 5–7; role-making, 5–6

Pennell, Marryland, 47

Personhood, risks to in medical training, 25–27

Peterson, Franklynn, 82

Physicians: divorce among, 3; health problems, ix–x; interaction with patients, 97–98

*Pre-Med Journal*, 16, 23

Presentation of self. *See* Facework

Private life: influence on career choices, 80–83, 102; inundation by training, 1–3, 58, 101–108

Professional calling: compromises in, 82–83, 103–106; service orientation, 106

Profession of medicine: heresy within, ix, 72, 107–108; responsibilities of, 77; rewards of, 107–108; sexism within, 88–91

Professionalism: ideology of, 5; tempering influence of, 108–111

Professional demeanor, problems of, 48–49

Professional identity: internalization of, 36–38; presentation of, 29–30

Professional socialization: assumptions about, 11–12; impact on private life, 11–13; literature on, 3–5; meaning of, 4–5; neglected areas of study, 3–4; punishment-centered, 102; purposes of, 4; status passage to adulthood, 101. *See also* Medical training

Qualitative methodology. *See* Research methodology

Research methodology, 5–11; constant comparison, 8; interviewing, 7–9; negotiating roles, 6; sampling, 6–9; theoretical coding, 9–11

Residencies, demands of, 76–77

Rist, Ray C., 5

Ritzer, George, 114

Role-taking, 85

Rose, K. Daniel, 3

Rosenberg, Mark L., 58

Rosow, Irving, 3

Ruzek, Sheryl K., 90–91

Safilios-Rothschild, Constantina, 114

Schatzman, Leonard, 114

Schutz, Alfred, 2, 113

Scott, Marvin B., 113–114

Shaffir, William, 29

Shapiro, Martin, 11, 17, 29, 58, 110, 114

Shibutani, Tamotsu, 38, 40

Skipper, James K., 80

Slowell, Shirlene, 47

Smith, Burke M., 63

Stelling, Joan G., 113

Stone, Gregory P., 18–19, 38, 52

Strauss, Anselm L., 8, 10–12, 19, 35, 38, 40, 55, 80, 99, 114

Student Health Organization, 87

Symbolic articulation, process of, 37, 40

Taylor, Steven J., 114
Training situation: multiplicity of, 86–87, 98–100; students adjustment to, 85–86; students influence on, 85–100. *See also* Medical schools
Travisano, Richard V., 36–37
Trice, Harrison M., 114
Tringo, John L., 39
Truman, Stanley R., 44
Turner, Ralph, 85

Unruh, David R., 99
U.S. Dept. of Health, Education, and Welfare, 3–4, 53, 114

Vincent, Clark E., 4, 113

Warkov, Seymour, 113

Wertz, Dorothy C., 90
Wertz, Richard W., 90
Whittaker, Elvi W., 3, 5, 113
Whyte, William Foote, 6
Woman, identity of, 39
Women: as applicants, 21–27; medical theories of, 88–91; as patients, 89
Women's Health Perspective, 88–91
Women Medical Students: adaptation to training, 50–52; being single, 51; discrimination of, 72; needs of, 95–96; percentage of, 47; problems of, 48–52, support groups, 97

Zabarenko, Lucy M., 36
Zabarenko, Ralph N., 36
Zelan, Joseph, 113
Zola, Irving, 89